Sexually Transmitted Diseases

Recent Titles in
A&A Health Guides

Self-Injury: Your Questions Answered
Romeo Vitelli

Living Green: Your Questions Answered
Amy Hackney Blackwell

SEXUALLY TRANSMITTED DISEASES

Your Questions Answered

Paul Quinn

Q&A Health Guides

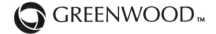

An Imprint of ABC-CLIO, LLC

Santa Barbara, California • Denver, Colorado

Library of Congress Cataloging-in-Publication Data

Names: Quinn, Paul, 1971– author.
Title: Sexually transmitted diseases : your questions answered / Paul Quinn.
Description: Santa Barbara, California : Greenwood, an imprint of ABC-CLIO, LLC,
    [2018] | Series: Q&A health guides | Includes bibliographical references and index.
Identifiers: LCCN 2017046441 (print) | LCCN 2017048727 (ebook) |
    ISBN 9781440853173 (ebook) | ISBN 9781440853166 (print : alk. paper)
Subjects: LCSH: Sexually transmitted diseases.
Classification: LCC RA644.V4 (ebook) | LCC RA644.V4 Q87 2018 (print) |
    DDC 616.95—dc23
LC record available at https://lccn.loc.gov/2017046441

ISBN: 978-1-4408-5316-6 (print)
      978-1-4408-5317-3 (eBook)

22 21 20 19 18   1 2 3 4 5

This book is also available as an eBook.

Greenwood
An Imprint of ABC-CLIO, LLC

ABC-CLIO, LLC
130 Cremona Drive, P.O. Box 1911
Santa Barbara, California 93116–1911
www.abc-clio.com

This book is printed on acid-free paper ∞

Manufactured in the United States of America

For Mom and David

Contents

Series Foreword   xi

Acknowledgments   xiii

Introduction   xv

Guide to Health Literacy   xvii

Common Misconceptions about STDs   xxv

Questions and Answers   1

General Information   3

    1. What is an STD?   3
    2. Is there a difference between an STD and a sexually
       transmitted infection (STI)?   4
    3. How many STDs occur in the United States each year?   6
    4. Which STDs are the most common?   7
    5. Are there different types of STDs?   8
    6. Are there different STDs for men and women?   10
    7. Do STDs only happen to young people?   11
    8. If I practice anal sex, am I still at risk for STDs?   12
    9. What are the risks associated with homosexual sex?   14
    10. Does being transgender affect my chances of
       contracting an STD?   15

11. Can I still get pregnant in the future if I had an STD?   16
12. Can an STD be transmitted to my baby if I get pregnant?   18
13. If neither one of us has an orgasm, can we still get
     an STD?   21
14. If I had an STD in the past, will it show up on
     a physical exam or in a blood test later?   22

Different Types of STDs   25

15. What is chlamydia?   25
16. What is gonorrhea?   29
17. What is trichomoniasis?   33
18. What are genital herpes?   35
19. What are genital warts?   41
20. What is syphilis?   45
21. What is Hepatitis B?   52
22. What is Hepatitis C?   55
23. What is HIV?   59
24. What is bacterial vaginosis?   71
25. What are "water warts"?   75
26. What is chancroid?   78
27. What is HPV?   82
28. What is pelvic inflammatory disease?   85
29. What is mucopurulent cervicitis?   88
30. What is lymphogranuloma venereum?   90
31. Is a yeast infection an STD?   93
32. Can men get a yeast infection?   96
33. What are "crabs"?   98
34. What are scabies?   101

Signs, Symptoms, and Diagnosis   105

35. Does everyone always develop symptoms of an STD?   105
36. What are the most common signs and symptoms
     of an STD?   106
37. Can I be tested for an STD and how?   107
38. How soon can I be tested for an STD after having
     unprotected sex?   108
39. Is there a test for every STD?   110
40. Can I tell if someone has an STD before having sex
     with them?   111

Treatment and Prevention 113

    41. What should I do if I think I have an STD? 113
    42. What can happen if an STD isn't treated? 114
    43. Does my partner have to be treated if I have an STD? Or do I have to get treatment if my partner has an STD but I feel OK? 115
    44. Can I treat an STD on my own naturally or with over-the-counter medication? 117
    45. Are STDs preventable? 119
    46. Does douching after sex minimize my chances of getting an STD? 120
    47. Do lubricants or spermicides decrease my chances of contracting an STD? 121
    48. Is there anything I can do through diet, exercise, or taking supplements to minimize my chances of getting an STD? 122
    49. Can STDs be transmitted through oral sex? 124
    50. If I have an STD, am I contagious? 126
    51. Do uncircumcised men transmit STDs more? 128

Case Studies 131

Glossary 145

Directory of Resources 147

Index 151

About the Author 155

Series Foreword

All of us have questions about our health. Is this normal? Should I be doing something differently? Who should I talk to about my concerns? And our modern world is full of answers. Thanks to the Internet, there's a wealth of information at our fingertips, from forums where people can share their personal experiences to Wikipedia articles to the full text of medical studies. But finding the right information can be an intimidating and difficult task—some sources are written at too high a level, others have been oversimplified, while still others are heavily biased or simply inaccurate.

Q&A Health Guides address the needs of readers who want accurate, concise answers to their health questions, authored by reputable and objective experts, and written in clear and easy-to-understand language. This series focuses on the topics that matter most to young adult readers, including various aspects of physical and emotional well-being, as well as other components of a healthy lifestyle. These guides will also serve as a valuable tool for parents, school counselors, and others who may need to answer teens' health questions.

All books in the series follow the same format to make finding information quick an easy. Each volume begins with an essay on health literacy and why it is so important when it comes to gathering and evaluating health information. Next, the top five myths and misconceptions that surround the topic are dispelled. The heart of each guide is a collection of questions and answers, organized thematically. A selection of five case studies provides real-world examples to illuminate key concepts. Rounding out each volume is a directory of resources, glossary, and index.

It is our hope that the books in this series will not only provide valuable information but will also help guide readers toward a lifetime of healthy decision making.

Acknowledgments

This work would not be possible without the support and encourage-ment from my family, friends, and colleagues. Specifically, sincere thanks and appreciation to Eileen Guidice, David Gilsenan, "Maggie," Tina Neri-Badame, Gregory Locoparra, Denise Mojica, Mary Quinn, Kelly Greco, John and Mindy Gilsenan, Mike and Mary Lanni, Christine Lanni, Michael Lanni and Alyssa DeJoy, John and Gina Nicoletti-Gilsenan, Kate and Marwan Amaisse, Matt Gilsenan, and the late Gladys Gilsenan. Additionally, Maryanne Hedrick, Alex Keomurjian, Larry Lane, Joel Kunkel, Jim McCoy, Ian Klein, and the "Boys of 96 Teal" were in my corner to cheer me on to complete this book.

Creating this book would not have been possible without key people who worked with me to inspire the idea, make necessary connections, and develop ideas. I am extremely grateful to Anthony Chiffolo, Maxine Taylor, and Lettie Conrad for their literary and publishing expertise and direction.

Inspiration comes in many forms, so I remain forever grateful to the thousands of men and women whom I had the privilege to care for, and care about, as my patients over two decades of nursing and midwifery practice. They, above all else, inspire me. Thank you for sharing your lives and stories with me that left a permanent mark within my soul.

Introduction

Sexually transmitted diseases (STDs) are on the rise globally. Regardless of advances in science, technology, or pharmaceuticals, an estimated 19.7 million STDs are diagnosed each year in the United States alone. This translates, then, to mean that approximately 1 out of 4 teens will contract an STD, or 1 out of 2 sexually active persons, overall, will contract an STD by age 25. These staggering statistics, then, demonstrate the need for the development of targeted tactics to reduce the overall incidence and prevalence of STDs internationally.

Education has been highlighted as a key strategy toward reducing, or eliminating, STDs. In the modern age, the explosion of information available on the Internet has been both a benefit and a hindrance to combatting STDs. On one hand, there is an abundance of information available if one were to explore an STD or a set of specific symptoms. Conversely, not all the information on the Internet is factual, accurate, or applicable to specific diseases or symptoms. Further, the suggestions for care, treatment, or prevention are often vague, doing little to reduce the fear or stigma associated with actual or potential STDs.

The purpose of this book, then, is to provide information, and education, in a simple format regarding each of the individual STDs, their signs or symptoms, and potential treatment plan. STDs carry an unnecessary fear or stigma for the person, or partner(s), impacted by one. The time has arrived to abolish those sentiments and refocus the emphasis of STDs toward prevention, early identification, control of transmission, and the development of an individualized, comprehensive treatment plan. This book, then, answers the questions many people are afraid, or embarrassed, to ask using the most recent, accurate, scientific evidence available in easy-to-understand language.

Guide to Health Literacy

On her 13th birthday, Samantha was diagnosed with type 2 diabetes. She consulted her mom and her aunt, both of whom also have type 2 diabetes and decided to go with their strategy of managing diabetes by taking insulin. As a result of participating in an after-school program at her middle school that focused on health literacy, she learned that she can help manage the level of glucose in her bloodstream by counting her carbohydrate intake, following a diabetic diet, and exercising regularly. But, what exactly should she do? How does she keep track of her carbohydrate intake? What is a diabetic diet? How long should she exercise and what type of exercise should she do? Samantha is a visual learner, so she turned to her favorite source of media, YouTube, to answer these questions. She found videos from individuals around the world sharing their experiences and tips, doctors (or at least people who have "Dr." in their YouTube channel names), government agencies such as the National Institutes of Health, and even video clips from cat lovers who have cats with diabetes. With guidance from the librarian and the health and science teachers at her school, she assessed the credibility of the information in these videos and even compared their suggestions to some of the print resources that she was able to find at her school library. Now, she knows exactly how to count her carbohydrate level, how to prepare and follow a diabetic diet, and how much (and what) exercise is needed daily. She intends to share her findings with her mom and her aunt, and now she wants to create a chart that summarizes what she has learned that she can share with her doctor.

Samantha's experience is not unique. She represents a shift in our society; an individual no longer views himself or herself as a passive recipient of medical care but as an active mediator of his or her own health. However, in this era when any individual can post his or her opinions and experiences with a particular health condition online with just a few clicks or publish a memoir, it is vital that people know how to assess the credibility of health information. Gone are the days when "publishing" health information required intense vetting. The health information landscape is highly saturated, and people have innumerable sources where they can find information about practically any health topic. The sources (whether print, online, or a person) that an individual consults for health information are crucial because the accuracy and trustworthiness of the information can potentially affect his or her overall health. The ability to find, select, assess, and use health information constitutes a type of literacy—health literacy—that everyone must possess.

THE DEFINITION AND PHASES OF HEALTH LITERACY

One of the most popular definitions for health literacy comes from Ratzan and Parker (2000), who describe health literacy as "the degree to which individuals have the capacity to obtain, process, and understand basic health information and services needed to make appropriate health decisions." Recent research has extrapolated health literacy into health literacy bits, further shedding light on the multiple phases and literacy practices that are embedded within the multifaceted concept of health literacy. Although this research has focused primarily on online health information seeking, these health literacy bits are needed to successfully navigate both print and online sources. There are six phases of health information seeking: (1) information need identification and question formulation, (2) information search, (3) information comprehension, (4) information assessment, (5) information management, and (6) information use.

The first phase is the *information need identification and question formulation phase*. In this phase, one needs to be able to develop and refine a range of questions to frame one's search and understand relevant health terms. In the second phase, *information search*, one has to possess appropriate searching skills, such as using proper keywords and correct spelling in search terms, especially when using search engines and databases. It is also crucial to understand how search engines work (i.e., how search results are derived, what the order of the search results means, how to use the snippets that are provided in the search results list to select websites, and how to determine which listings are ads on a search engine results page). One also has to limit reliance on surface characteristics, such as the design of a website or a book (a website or book that appears to have a lot of information or looks aesthetically pleasant does not necessarily mean it has good information) and language used (a website or book that utilizes jargon, the keywords that one used to conduct the search, or the word "information" does not necessarily indicate it will have good information). The next phase is *information comprehension*, whereby one needs to have the ability to read, comprehend, and recall the information (including textual, numerical, and visual content) one has located from the books and/or online resources.

To assess the credibility of health information (*information assessment* phase), one needs to be able to evaluate information for accuracy, evaluate how current the information is (e.g., when a website was last updated or when a book was published), and evaluate the creators of the source—for example, examine site sponsors or type of sites (.com, .gov, .edu, or .org) or the author of a book (practicing doctor, a celebrity doctor, a patient of a specific disease, etc.) to determine the believability of the person/organization providing the information. Such credibility perceptions tend to become generalized, so they must be frequently reexamined (e.g., the belief that a specific news agency always has credible health information needs continuous vetting). One also needs to evaluate the credibility of the medium (e.g., television, Internet, radio, social media, and book) and evaluate—not just accept without questioning—others' claims regarding the validity of a site, book, or other specific source of information. At this stage, one has to "make sense of information gathered from diverse sources by identifying misconceptions, main and supporting ideas, conflicting information, point of view, and biases" (American Association of School Librarians [AASL], 2009, p. 13) and conclude which sources/information are valid and accurate by using conscious strategies rather than simply using intuitive judgments or "rules of thumb." This phase is the most challenging segment of health information seeking and serves as a determinant of success (or lack thereof) in the information-seeking process. The following section on Sources of Health Information further explains this phase.

The fifth phase is *information management*, whereby one has to organize information that has been gathered in some manner to ensure easy retrieval and use in the future. The last phase is *information use*, in which one will synthesize information found across various resources, draw conclusions, and locate the answer to his or her original question and/or the content that fulfills the information need. This phase also often involves implementation, such as using the information to solve a health problem; make health-related decisions; identify and engage in behaviors that will help a person to avoid health risks; share the health information found with family members and friends who may benefit from it; and advocate more broadly for personal, family, or community health.

THE IMPORTANCE OF HEALTH LITERACY

The conception of health has moved from a passive view (someone is either well or ill) to one that is more active and process based (someone is working toward preventing or managing disease). Hence, the dominant focus has shifted from doctors and treatments to patients and prevention, resulting in the need to strengthen our ability and confidence (as patients and consumers of health care) to look for, assess, understand, manage, share, adapt, and use health-related information. An individual's health literacy level has been found to predict his or her health status better than age, race, educational attainment, employment status, and income level (National Network of Libraries of Medicine [NNLM], 2013). Greater health literacy also enables individuals to better communicate with health-care providers such as doctors, nutritionists, and therapists, as they can pose more relevant, informed, and useful questions to health-care providers. Another added advantage of greater health literacy is better information-seeking skills not only for health but also in other domains, such as completing assignments for school.

SOURCES OF HEALTH INFORMATION: THE GOOD, THE BAD, AND THE IN-BETWEEN

For generations, doctors, nurses, nutritionists, health coaches, and other health professionals have been the trusted sources of health information. Additionally, researchers have found that young adults, when they have health-related questions, typically turn to a family member who has had firsthand experience with a health condition because of their family member's close proximity and because of their past experience with, and trust in, this individual. Expertise should be a core consideration when consulting a person, website, or book for health information. The credentials and background of the person or author and conflicting interests of the author (and his or her organization) must be checked and validated to ensure the likely credibility of the health information they are conveying. While books often have implied credibility because of the peer-review process involved, self-publishing has challenged this credibility, so qualifications of book authors should also be verified. When it comes to health information, currency of the source must also be examined. When examining health information/studies presented, pay attention to the exhaustiveness of research methods utilized to offer recommendations or conclusions. Small and nondiverse sample size is often—but not always—an indication of reduced credibility. Studies that confuse correlation with causation is another potential issue to watch for. Information seekers must also pay attention to the sponsors of the research studies. For example, if a study is sponsored by manufacturers of drug Y and the study recommends that drug Y is the best treatment to manage or cure a disease, this may indicate a lack of objectivity on the part of the researchers.

The Internet is rapidly becoming one of the main sources of health information. Online forums, news agencies, personal blogs, social media sites, pharmacy sites, and celebrity "doctors" are all offering medical and health information targeted to various types of people in regard to all types of diseases and symptoms. There are professional journalists, citizen journalists, hoaxers, and people paid to write fake health news on various sites that may appear to have a legitimate domain name and may even have authors who claim to have professional credentials, such as an MD. All these sites *may* offer useful information or information that appears to be useful and relevant; however, much of the information may be debatable and may fall into gray areas that require readers to discern credibility, reliability, and biases.

While broad recognition and acceptance of certain media, institutions, and people often serve as the most popular determining factors to assess credibility of health information among young people, keep in mind that there are legitimate Internet sites, databases, and books that publish health information and serve as sources of health information for doctors, other health sites, and members of the public. For example, MedlinePlus (https://medlineplus.gov) has trusted sources on over 975 diseases and conditions and presents the information in easy-to-understand language.

The chart here presents factors to consider when assessing credibility of health information. However, keep in mind that these factors function only as a guide and require continuous updating to keep abreast with the changes in the landscape of health information, information sources, and technologies.

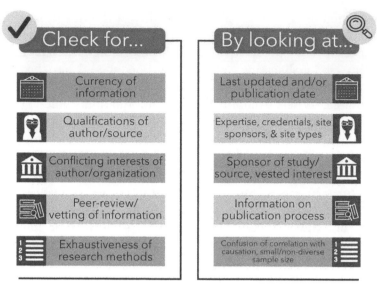

All images from flaticon.com

The chart can serve as a guide; however, approaching a librarian about how one can go about assessing the credibility of both print and online health information is far more effective than using generic checklist-type tools. While librarians are not health experts, they can apply and teach patrons strategies to determine the credibility of health information.

With the prevalence of fake sites and fake resources that appear to be legitimate, it is important to use the following health information assessment tips to verify health information that one has obtained (St. Jean et al., 2015, p. 151):

- **Don't assume you are right:** Even when you feel very sure about an answer, keep in mind that the answer may not be correct, and it is important to conduct (further) searches to validate the information.
- **Don't assume you are wrong:** You may actually have correct information, even if the information you encounter does not match—that is, you may be right and the resources that you have found may contain false information.
- **Take an open approach:** Maintain a critical stance by not including your preexisting beliefs as keywords (or letting them influence your choice of keywords) in a search, as this may influence what it is possible to find out.
- **Verify, verify, and verify:** Information found, especially on the Internet, needs to be validated, no matter how the information appears on

the site (i.e., regardless of the appearance of the site or the quantity of information that is included).

Health literacy comes with experience navigating health information. Professional sources of health information, such as doctors, health-care providers, and health databases, are still the best, but one also has the power to search for health information and then verify it by consulting with these trusted sources and by using the health information assessment tips and guide shared previously.

Mega Subramaniam, PhD
Associate Professor, College of Information Studies,
University of Maryland

REFERENCES AND FURTHER READING

American Association of School Librarians (AASL). (2009). *Standards for the 21st-century learner in action.* Chicago, IL: American Association of School Librarians.

Hilligoss, B., & Rieh, S. Y. (2008). Developing a unifying framework of credibility assessment: Construct, heuristics, and interaction in context. *Information Processing & Management, 44*(4), 1467–1484.

Kuhlthau, C. C. (1988). Developing a model of the library search process: Cognitive and affective aspects. *Reference Quarterly, 28*(2), 232–242.

National Network of Libraries of Medicine (NNLM). (2013). *Health literacy.* Bethesda, MD: National Network of Libraries of Medicine. Retrieved from nnlm.gov/outreach/consumer/hlthlit.html.

Ratzan, S. C., & Parker, R. M. (2000). Introduction. In C. R. Selden, M. Zorn, S. C. Ratzan, & R. M. Parker (eds.), *National Library of Medicine current bibliographies in medicine: Health literacy.* NLM Pub. No. CBM 2000–1. Bethesda, MD: National Institutes of Health, U.S. Department of Health and Human Services.

St. Jean, B., Taylor, N. G., Kodama, C., & Subramaniam, M. (2017, February). Assessing the health information source perceptions of tweens using card-sorting exercises. *Journal of Information Science.* Retrieved from http://journals.sagepub.com/doi/abs/10.1177/0165551516687728.

St. Jean, B., Subramaniam, M., Taylor, N. G., Follman, R., Kodama, C., & Casciotti, D. (2015). The influence of positive hypothesis testing on youths' online health-related information seeking. *New Library World, 116*(3/4), 136–154.

Subramaniam, M., St. Jean, B., Taylor, N.G., Kodama, C., Follman, R., & Casciotti, D. (2015). Bit by bit: Using design-based research to improve the health literacy of adolescents. *JMIR Research Protocols*, 4(2), paper e62. Retrieved from www.ncbi.nlm.nih.gov/pmc/articles/PMC4464334/.

Valenza, J. (2016, November 26). Truth, truthiness, and triangulation: A news literacy toolkit for a "post-truth" world [Web log]. Retrieved from http://blogs.slj.com/neverendingsearch/2016/11/26/truth-truthi ness-triangulation-and-the-librarian-way-a-news-literacy-toolkit-for-a-post-truth-world/.

Common Misconceptions
about STDs

1. STDs ONLY HAPPEN TO PROMISCUOUS PEOPLE

Anyone who is sexually active is at risk for contracting an STD. While oral, vaginal, or anal sex with multiple different partners increases a person's risk of contracting an STD, any of the STDs can be transmitted from an infected person to an uninfected partner with even a brief, singular sexual encounter. All that is necessary, then, to transmit the microorganisms that cause STDs is unprotected (i.e., not using a male or female condom) oral, vaginal, or anal sexual intercourse. During unprotected sexual intercourse, any disease-causing microorganisms can enter an uninfected person's body through breaks in the skin and mucous membranes or by skin-to-skin contact for certain specific organisms. The proper and consistent use of barrier methods, such as the male or female condom, then, is currently the most effective way to prevent transmitting STDs between partners during any episode of sexual activity. For more information about the incidence of STDs, refer to Questions 3 and 4.

2. STDs ONLY HAPPEN TO GIRLS

STDs occur in both men and women. While women are more susceptible to a host of diseases that are unique only to women because of the anatomical structures of the female genital area or the presence of female pelvic organs like the cervix, uterus, or fallopian tubes (e.g., bacterial vaginosis, pelvic inflammatory disease, or mucopurulent cervicitis), both men and women alike share equal susceptibility to contracting an STD from sexual activity. STDs, then, do not discriminate between men and women. Additionally, both men and women share the ability to prevent transmitting or contracting STDs through the proper and consistent use of condoms as barrier methods and by participating in regular STD screenings to identify the presence of any STDs, and allow treatment to be initiated, sooner. For more information on specific STDs for both men and women, refer to Question 6.

3. MEN CANNOT TRANSMIT STDs

Both men and women, if infected with the microorganisms that cause specific STDs, can easily transmit an infection to an uninfected partner during sexual activity. During episodes of unprotected sexual activity (i.e., sex without a condom), the penis is in direct contact with the lining, or mucous membranes, of the mouth, vagina, or anus. Seminal fluid (i.e., "pre-cum") or semen, then, can further coat these internal surfaces and expand the amount of surface area of vulnerable tissues that can be exposed to harmful bacteria, viruses, fungus, or protozoans that might be growing, or thriving, in a man's body fluids. Repeated episodes of sexual intercourse or activity, then, increases the risk of uninfected male or female sex partners to contract an STD transmitted by an infected male. The proper and consistent use of condoms, then, serves as the most effective way for men to prevent transmitting harmful, STD-causing microorganisms to their sex partners. For more information on transmission of each individual STD, refer to Questions 15 through 33.

4. STDs ALWAYS HAVE WIDESPREAD SYSTEMIC EFFECTS ON THE BODY

Most STDs that are diagnosed early, and successfully treated or managed, have minimal effects on the organ systems of the body. What determines the likelihood of a specific STD causing harm to other organ systems of the body is whether the STD is bacterial, viral, fungal, or protozoan in nature and the amount of time the disease has been active within the body prior to being diagnosed. In general, the longer an STD is left untreated the more likely it is to cause harm or damage to the organs of the body. Most bacterial STDs (i.e., gonorrhea or chlamydia) respond well to a course of antibiotic therapy that successfully eradicates the disease. An STD like syphilis, in contrast, may go undiagnosed in its earlier stage and, therefore, cause damage to specific organs within the body over time. Similarly, viral STDs such as herpes or HIV are not curable with current antiviral therapies; the viruses which cause illness lie dormant within the body and continue to weaken structures or organ systems over time with each subsequent disease flare-up. Additionally, untreated STDs may also interfere with a man or woman's fertility, or a woman's ability to sustain a pregnancy. It is essential, then, for sexually active people to participate in regular follow-up with a health-care practitioner where STD screenings can be used to identify the presence of STDs sooner. For more information on STD testing, diagnosis, treatment, and systemic effects, refer to Questions 11, 12, 14, 34 through 38, and 41 through 43.

5. ANY VAGINAL OR PENILE COMPLAINT WITH PAIN, MALODOROUS DISCHARGE, OR ITCHING IS ALWAYS AN STD

Many STDs have no symptoms at the onset. Often as an STD remains undiagnosed and continues to advance, symptoms may develop which classically include penile or vaginal discharge, pain, burning or itching, alone or in combination. The classic STD symptoms, however, are also indicative of other conditions (e.g., kidney stone, urinary tract infection, injury) that are unrelated to an STD. The only way to determine the cause of any penile or vaginal symptoms, then, is to obtain a comprehensive evaluation from a health-care practitioner with STD screening if indicated. Similarly, one should not automatically assume any genital symptoms indicate an STD, forego an evaluation or treatment by a health-care practitioner, and opt instead to "ride it out," "let it pass," or attempt to self-treat any condition. An evaluation by a health-care practitioner, then, remains the safest, most effective way to properly diagnose and treat the causes of any genital symptoms. For more information on STD symptoms and treatments, refer to Questions 15 through 33, 39, and 42 through 47.

QUESTIONS AND ANSWERS

General Information

1. What is an STD?

Sexually transmitted diseases (STDs) are any number of infections, conditions, or diseases that occur as a direct result of sex, sexual activity, or intimate contact with a partner. Because the genital areas of both males and females are typically a warm, moist environment, there is a proliferation of various viruses, bacteria, protozoa, and fungi. These microorganisms, then, can survive indefinitely on both the skin surfaces of the genital areas and within the mucous membranes (i.e., the surfaces inside the vagina, penis, or rectum) regardless of a person's hygiene or health habits. While a majority of these microorganisms are harmless, some can be disease-causing. These disease-causing organisms, then, can be passed easily from person to person through semen, vaginal and other body fluids, blood, or by direct skin-to-skin contact. What makes STDs so problematic, and such a public health concern, is that these diseases can be transmitted from people who seem perfectly healthy and who may not even be aware they have an infection at all. The only common factor, however, that STDs share is that they are transmitted through some sort of sexual activity or intimate contact.

Sexual activity is on the rise throughout the United States and among the developed nations throughout the world. Greater than 60 percent of teens report engaging in some form of sexual activity before the age of 17, and more than 45 percent of teens reported regular sexual intercourse with different partners during their high school years. Among young adults in the age range of 20 to 30 years, more than 80 percent reported engaging in regular sexual activity, often with different partners outside a traditional monogamous relationship. A more impressive statistic is that 51 percent of people engaging in sexual activity in the United States reported practicing unprotected sex. Not surprising, then, the Centers for Disease Control and Prevention (CDC) estimates that nearly 20 million new sexually transmitted infections occur every year in the United States, half among young people aged 15 to 24. Despite the high incidence of STDs in the United States, few, if any, are fatal and most are preventable. While each infection is a potential threat to an individual's immediate and long-term health and well-being, most STDs are treatable once diagnosed.

2. Is there a difference between an STD and a sexually transmitted infection (STI)?

The term "STD" is often used interchangeably with "sexually transmitted infection" (STI). The amount of information available in print or electronically where STD and STI are either used interchangeably or in combination can be overwhelming and confusing. There is a difference between the two terms; the difference, however, depends upon the source of the information.

If the information is coming from any of the health sciences, for example, items written by physicians or nurses, the term "STI" is often used to delineate people who have come in contact with any of the microorganisms that can cause a sexually transmitted illness or condition. Despite coming in contact with those microorganisms, the person has no outward signs or symptoms that suggest he or she may have active disease. Since there are no symptoms, the person has no reason to seek medical care or screening. However, the person is still capable of passing those microorganisms to a sex partner during sexual activity. What is important to keep in mind is that while one person without symptoms of a sexually transmitted illness or condition passed on microorganisms to his or her partner, symptoms can easily, and quickly, develop in his or her now-infected sex partner.

Similarly, the terms "STI" and "STD" are often used for specific types of infections depending on their severity and duration. For example, gonorrhea has specific signs and symptoms that, once experienced, can compel someone to seek medical care, screening, and appropriate treatment.

Treatment is typically effective, where the bacterium that caused gonor-rhea is destroyed, the person's symptoms clear, and there are no long-term effects or consequences. Gonorrhea, then, is often referred to as an STI because it is a short-lived condition that can be effectively eliminated without lifelong consequences. STIs, then, are often considered similar to other infections that a person may experience at any time in his or her lives such as strep throat, "pink eye," or the common cold: episodic, time-limited, and treatable.

Conversely, the term "STD" is often used for conditions where the microorganisms acquired during sexual activity lead to an infection and, as a consequence of contracting that infection, a lifelong condition remains. Even though a treatment for the specific infection is available and removes the immediate signs and symptoms of that infection, the person is never fully cured and will always carry the risk of the illness, or infection, flaring up and needing another course of treatment. Further, these specific conditions can be spread easily from partner to partner with sexual activity, even if there are no obvious signs and symptoms of an infection. For example, genital herpes begins as an infection in the geni-tal area that is spread during sexual activity with a partner who is already infected with the virus that causes genital herpes. The infected person can shed the virus that is easily passed on to a sex partner, even if the infected person has no outward signs or symptoms of an impending flare up or out-break. Once an active herpes infection occurs, painful lesions erupt in the genital area that can be treated with a regimen of antiviral medication. Even though the lesions subside and there is no longer obvious infection, for the rest of that person's life he or she will always have the virus that causes genital herpes lying dormant within his or her body. At times, that virus can awaken and cause flare ups or recurrent outbreaks. Because gen-ital herpes is permanent, it is frequently referred to as an STD instead of a simple infection.

Because calling some conditions infections and others diseases can be confusing or misleading, many experts often utilize one consistent term when describing the myriad of conditions or illnesses that occur due to sexual activity. Calling these conditions or illnesses "diseases," then, is the traditional term that is used, and understood, by many. Further, the initials "STD" have a time-honored understanding to capture all of those conditions, illnesses, or infections that result from sexual activity. While many groups have tried to minimize the stigma of STDs by calling them STIs, the majority of sexually active people identify and understand the term "STD" to encompass all of the conditions that may be transmitted through sexual activity. Further, many experts contest that calling certain diseases infections and other diseases minimizes the importance of overall sexual health and responsible sexual activity by classifying some conditions as potentially minor or easily fixable. The incorrect message, then, is that some infections are less serious or problematic, while only those with lifelong consequences are critical or devastating.

While the experts differ on the terminology of these conditions, all agree that any sexually transmitted condition can have serious, long-term consequences. Because these consequences are common and potentially dangerous or life-altering, most experts will continue to use the term "STD" to classify these conditions. The message that is consistent among all the experts is that STDs are preventable, with most treatable and controllable. Proper screening and health care, then, are the essential components of minimizing any consequences that can occur as a result of specific STDs, along with minimizing the transmission of any STDs to someone else.

3. How many STDs occur in the United States each year?

According to the CDC, approximately 110 million Americans have an STD at any given time. Further, in the United States nearly 20 million cases of new or first time STDs are reported each year. However, these numbers can be misleading because the numbers reported rely on STDs that were actually diagnosed; a significant portion of the population is currently infected with some form of STD and is unaware they have a disease that they can spread easily to others. The overall number of STDs in the United States, then, is actually higher than the current CDC estimates.

Capturing the total number of STDs in the United States, however, is difficult. The data available are based on state and local STD case reports that come from various public and private sources. The main source of the cases reported, then, is non-STD clinic settings such as private physician offices and health maintenance organizations. Not all cases of STDs, then, are captured and reported through state and local reporting mechanisms; only select STDs are required to be reported. Further, some cases of STDs were secondary diagnoses to conditions with other similar symptoms and therefore not treated, or captured, as the primary diagnosis. Similarly, several STDs, such as human papillomavirus (HPV), herpes simplex virus (HSV), and trichomoniasis, are not routinely reported to the CDC, adding to the difficulty of obtaining a complete, or total, number of STDs occurring annually. Because of the inconsistencies in reporting for STDs overall, only a fraction of the true volume of STDs in the United States can be estimated. Regardless, the estimated numbers are impressive and compelling in regard to the prevalence, incidence, and trends in STDs across the United States.

The growing number of new STD cases in the United States demonstrates that STDs are a significant health-care challenge in the nation. STDs not only increase a person's risk for acquiring and transmitting human immunodeficiency virus (HIV) infection but also contribute to severe health complications such as infertility or ectopic pregnancy. Additionally, more than half of the reported cases of STDs are occurring in young people aged 15 to 24. Each STD, then, is a potential threat to a person's immediate health that could have devastating, lifelong consequences to a person's health and well-being.

4. Which STDs are the most common?

In order to calculate the incidence or prevalence rates for individual STDs, the CDC relies on accurately reported data from state health departments to compile its statistics. State health departments, in turn, rely on information that is reported through local health departments, clinics, and individual health-care practitioners. Only select STDs are reported. There are a variety of STDs (e.g., HPV or HSV), however, that occur each year where no information is available to capture their true incidence or prevalence rates.

From the data available, the CDC reported that the eight most common STDs are chlamydia, gonorrhea, Hepatitis B virus (HBV), genital herpes, HIV, HPV, syphilis, and trichomoniasis. In 2014, increases in the number of new cases of chlamydia, gonorrhea, and syphilis were reported nationally. Young people aged 15 to 24 and women are the most severely affected by STDs. However, the increasing rates among men contributed to the overall increase in reported diseases in 2014. The CDC, therefore, reported that in 2014:

Chlamydia: 1,441,789 cases reported, which was an increase of 2.8 percent from 2013. Rate per 100,000 people: 456.1

Gonorrhea: 350,062 cases reported, which was an increase of 5.1 percent from 2013. Rate per 100,000 people: 110.7

Syphilis (primary and secondary): 19,999 cases reported, which was an increase of 15.1 percent from 2013. Rate per 100,000 people: 6.3

Syphilis (congenital): 458 cases reported, which was an increase of 27.5 percent from 2013. Rate per 100,000 live births: 11.6

While anyone can be infected with an STD, there are certain groups who are contracting STDs more frequently. Surveillance data demonstrates both the numbers and rates of reported cases of chlamydia and gonorrhea continue to be the highest among young people aged 15 to 24. While men and women are equally affected by STDs, young women face the most serious long-term health consequences. Conversely, men account for more than 90 percent of all primary and secondary syphilis cases reported in 2014. Further, men who have sex with men (MSM) account for 83 percent of male cases where the sex of the sex partner is known. Similarly, the available surveillance data indicate that averages of half the men who have sex with other men and have syphilis are also infected with HIV.

5. Are there different types of STDs?

There are many different types of STDs. It is easier, then, to understand the different types of STDs if they are broken down, or grouped, into families according to the causative microorganism: viral, bacterial, parasitic, and fungal.

Viral

Viral STDs are caused by viruses that are passed from person-to-person during sexual activity. Unlike other types of STDs, viral-based STDs are not localized to the genital area; their effects are systemic and involve different parts of the body at one time. Often there is no cure for viral STDs. Viral STDs include:

Human papillomavirus: The most common viral STD, HPV is actually a group of 150 related viruses, with 40 specific HPV types known to infect the male and female genital areas.

Genital herpes: Caused by the HSV, this virus is transmitted easily by sexual activities or skin-to-skin contact. HSV is part of the same family of viruses that cause cold sores in and around the mouth.

Hepatitis B virus: HBV is easily transmitted through sexual activity or by sharing items like razors, toothbrushes, or needles. HBV affects and can cause permanent damage to the liver.

Human immunodeficiency virus: HIV attacks the body's immune system, leaving an infected individual unable to fight off illnesses. It is transmitted through sexual activity but also spread by sharing items like razors, needles, or toothbrushes.

Bacterial

Bacterial STDs are caused by bacteria that are passed from person-to-person, typically during sexual activity. Symptoms of bacterial STDs can be vague or nonexistent. Most bacterial STDs can be successfully treated with antibiotics. Bacterial STDs include:

Chlamydia: One of the most common STDs, especially among people aged 15 to 24. If left untreated, it can cause infertility in both men and women.

Gonorrhea: An STD that is often transmitted at the same time as chlamydia, gonorrhea shares similar symptoms, if any, with chlamydia. It is not uncommon to treat someone for both chlamydia and gonorrhea at the same time if either one is suspected or found. Gonorrhea occurs most often in people aged 15 to 29. Left untreated, like chlamydia, gonorrhea can cause infertility in both men and women.

Syphilis: There are three stages of syphilis: primary, secondary, and latent or late stage. The primary stage starts with a small, painless sore where the bacteria entered the body. With secondary syphilis, a person may develop a general feeling of being ill or run down and find a flat, smooth wart or lesion in the genital area. In latent or late stage, syphilis, the untreated disease begins to damage other organs in the body such as the heart and brain and can cause death.

Parasitic

Parasitic STDs are caused by parasites (e.g., protozoa, mites, or insects) which are creatures that live off another body or host. The parasites are passed from person-to-person during sexual activity. Parasites, then, are similar or equivalent to small bugs that live off a human but cannot be seen by the naked eye. Parasites, however, are often able to be treated by specific medications. Parasitic STDs include:

Trichomoniasis: Caused by a single-celled protozoan, trichomoniasis is easily transmitted through sexual activity or sharing of sex toys. Trichomoniasis can infect the urethra in both men and women; the bladder, vagina, or cervix in women; or be found underneath the foreskin in men.

Pubic lice ("crabs"): Known as "crabs" because the lice insect resembles a small crab when visualized under a microscope, pubic lice live in the pubic hairs around the genitals. The lice cling to, and lay eggs, at the base of the hair.

Scabies: A disease caused by tiny mites that burrow under the top layers of the skin and lay eggs. The mites quickly mature and multiply, continuing to burrow and breed under the skin.

Fungal

While not technically STDs in most circumstances, fungal infections can be caused due to sexual activity or contact. Fungal infections are highly responsive to antifungal medications.

Yeast infection (vaginal candidiasis): A vaginal yeast infection is a common fungal infection caused by an overgrowth of naturally occurring yeast in the body, *Candida albicans*. Yeast is normally found in a woman's vagina in small numbers but, as new bacteria are introduced into the vagina during sex, the yeast can multiply and change the normal balance of bacteria within the vagina. When the overgrowth occurs, a fungal, or yeast, infection occurs.

6. Are there different STDs for men and women?

Each of the known STDs can affect men and women equally. However, women are more affected by STDs compared to men and disproportionately bear the long-term consequences of STDs. Further, the most serious long-term complications of STDs (i.e., pelvic inflammatory disease [PID], ectopic pregnancy, infertility, and chronic pelvic pain) only affect women. Where men and women differ, however, is how the various STDs affect each sex, with women, often, more severely impacted by STDs than men.

1. A woman's anatomy places her at a unique risk for STDs compared to a man. The inner lining of the vagina is thinner and more delicate than the skin of the penis, thereby making it easier for viruses or bacteria to penetrate the mucous membrane or skin surfaces. The vagina, further, is a moist environment that promotes, and sustains, the growth of microorganisms.
2. Women are less likely to have symptoms of common STDs such as chlamydia or gonorrhea compared to men. If symptoms do occur, they

can go away even though the infection may remain. Signs of infection within the vagina are difficult to visualize and therefore may go unnoticed or ignored.

3. Women are more likely to confuse symptoms of an STD for something else. Women often have vaginal discharge, for example, before a menstrual period, or mistake any burning or itching in the vaginal area for a yeast infection. Men, conversely, are often more aware of symptoms such as discharge because any symptoms, typically, are uncommon and unusual.

4. Women do not see signs of STDs as easily as men. Genital ulcers, for example, from herpes or syphilis, can occur in the vagina and may not be easily visible. Men, in contrast, will be more likely to notice sores or lesions since the penis and all its surfaces are easily visualized.

5. STDs can cause serious health complications that can affect a woman's future fertility. Untreated STDs can lead to PID which can, in turn, scar the fallopian tubes and cause ectopic pregnancies or infertility.

6. Women who are pregnant can pass STDs to their babies. Women can pass diseases such as genital herpes, syphilis, and HIV to their babies during pregnancy or at the time of delivery. STDs, further, can lead to miscarriages or stillbirths, blindness, deafness, brain damage, or cause babies to be born with a low birth weight.

7. Women who contract HPV are at higher risk of developing cervical cancer. While HPV is common in men, serious health problems rarely occur in men as a result of an HPV infection.

7. Do STDs only happen to young people?

STDs affect people of all ages. While people aged 15 to 24 accounts for half of all new STDs diagnosed, they represent just 25 percent of the sexually experienced population. The rates of STDs in middle-aged and older adults are rising. For example, recent statistics from the CDC have demonstrated that the number of new HIV infections is actually growing faster in individuals over age 50 than in people 40 years of age and younger. Additionally, the CDC also reported in 2010 that close to 2,550 cases of syphilis were reported among adults between the ages of 45 and 65, an increase from around 900 cases in 2000. Further, the number of reported chlamydia cases in the 45 to 65 age group tripled from nearly 6,700 cases in 2000 to 19,600 in 2010. There are multiple reasons, then, why STDs are impacting not only young people but also middle age and older adults.

Sexual activity occurs at any age. It is no surprise, then, that people in their 40s, 50s, 60s, 70s, and older, are having sex with long-term and new partners. Some adults in these age groups are ending previous relationships and dating again, while others have been single and enjoying various partners over time. People of all ages, then, participate in, and enjoy, sex and sexual activities. As such, the risks of contracting or transmitting STDs are the same for any person, regardless of age. Middle-aged and older adults, however, have different influences that impact their sexual practices. For example, there is an increased divorce rate currently in the United States. Consequently, middle-aged and older adults are returning to dating and experiencing both casual and long-term intimate or sexual relationships. The introduction of drugs for erectile dysfunction (e.g., Cialis, Levitra, or Viagra) and hormonal replacement for men have allowed middle-aged and older men to have the stamina and endurance necessary to enjoy, and sustain, sexual activity. Women, similarly, are remaining sexually active throughout adulthood and use both hormonal and nonhormonal supplements to maintain sexual drive and vitality. Additionally, middle-aged and older adults are freer to engage in bisexual and homosexual relationships.

While sexual activity, regardless of age, puts any person at risk for contracting or transmitting an STD, middle-aged and older adults face additional challenges because of age that puts them at increased risk for contracting an STD compared to younger people. For example, women who are postmenopausal often negate the need for contraceptives such as condoms since pregnancy is no longer a concern or an option. Additionally, as women age, the mucous membranes, and other surfaces of the vagina, lose their elasticity and natural lubrication. These tissues, then, become easily friable and susceptible to irritation, tears, and bleeding. These breaks in tissue, then, serve as a portal of entry for a host of microorganisms during sex. Similarly, middle age or older adults may not tolerate a rigorous course of antibiotic therapy as younger people, making it more difficult to treat specific STDs.

8. If I practice anal sex, am I still at risk for STDs?

Unprotected anal sex, regardless if it is practiced by hetero- or homosexual couples, is considered the riskiest activity for contracting and transmitting STDs because of the anatomy of the anus and the rectum. The anus is a tight, muscular band that easily constricts. Entry into the rectum, then, often requires force or pressure to pass through the anus. The rectum, further, is narrow and does not self-lubricate. The environment inside the rectum is warm and moist where bacterial infections such as chlamydia or gonorrhea can thrive. The skin and membranes of the anus and rectum are fragile and can tear easily, thereby providing portals of entry for micro-organisms such as HIV, HPV, or HBV to enter the bloodstream.

While unprotected anal sex is riskier for the receptive partner, the insertive partner (typically a male) is not free from risk. Both partners are susceptible to transmitting or contracting herpes, syphilis, and HPV. Con-dom use, while providing protection from a majority of STDs, does not fully minimize the risk of getting an STD with anal sex. Sores, lesions, or warts reside both inside and outside the anus and can be transmitting their causative virus through skin-to-skin contact or touching. Further, diseases like herpes can still be transmitted even if no genital lesions are present.

Anal sex makes a person susceptible to other conditions also. Since the lining of the anus and rectum is so fragile and tears easily, it also heals slowly once torn or damaged. Feces and fecal material that passes through the rectum and anus contain bacteria that can cause even small tears to become infected and possibly develop into an anal abscess. Because of the regular presence of feces and fecal matter in the rectum, the rectum is colonized with multiple microorganisms. For women, then, unprotected anal sex followed immediately by vaginal penetration brings all the harm-ful rectal microorganisms and introduces them directly into the vagina. While not a classic STD, severe, painful vaginal infections can develop that can cause numerous medical complications. The anal-to-vaginal sex pattern can also bring the harmful rectal microorganisms in contact with the urethra, or urinary opening, and contribute to the development of infections in the urinary tract and bladder.

Anal sex can still be practiced and enjoyed by both hetero- and homo-sexual couples with the risks of STDs or other infections minimized. While condoms do not provide complete protection against STDs related to anal sex, they continue to provide the best protection currently when used properly and consistently. There is more friction created during anal sex compared to vaginal sex, which can cause condoms to break. Using lubricant in sufficient quantities will not only protect the condom from breaking during anal sex but also prevent tears or breaks to the anus or rectal tissues or lining. Saliva should not be used as lubricant. Only water- or silicone-based lubricants should be used with latex condoms; oil-based lubricants such as baby oil, coconut oil, or petroleum jelly can damage condoms and cause them to break. Spermicidal creams used alone as lubri-cant can often be irritating to the rectum. Condoms should be changed regularly, especially before attempting vaginal penetration or oral sex.

9. What are the risks associated with homosexual sex?

Homosexual sex, where men have sex with men or women have sex with women, poses the same risks for transmitting and contracting STDs. Homosexual sex is not limited to gay men and lesbians. A growing number of people identify as heterosexual but participate in sexual activity with a same-sex partner. Men and women, however, have different risks associated with homosexual sex.

Men

The incidence of STDs has been increasing among gay and bisexual men, with increases in syphilis being seen across the United States. Gay, bisexual, and other MSM accounted for 83 percent of primary and secondary syphilis cases in 2014 where the sex of the sex partner was known. MSM are at risk for transmitting and contracting chlamydia, gonorrhea, and HPV. Some types of HPV, further, can cause genital or anal warts that could eventually develop into anal cancers. Gay, bisexual, and MSM are 15 to 17 times more likely to develop anal cancers compared to heterosexual men. Routinely practicing unprotected anal sex also increases a man's risk of contracting HIV and HBV.

Women

Lesbians, and women who have sex with women, are at risk for the same STDs as heterosexual women. STDs can be transmitted woman-to-woman by skin-to-skin contact, contact with vaginal mucous membranes, menstrual blood, or sharing sex toys. Two STDs are more common among lesbians and women who have sex with women: bacterial vaginosis (BV) and HPV.

While BV is not considered a classic STD, the microorganism that causes BV, *Gardnerella vaginalis*, or *G. vaginalis*, can be transmitted from woman to woman during sexual activity. BV, further, occurs more frequently among women who have recently acquired other STDs or had unprotected sex. For reasons that are unclear, BV is more common in lesbians and bisexual women compared to heterosexual women, and frequently occur in both members of lesbian couples. If left untreated, any woman with BV is susceptible to other STDs such as HIV, chlamydia, gonorrhea, and PID.

Lesbians, bisexual women, and women who have sex with other women can transmit HPV through direct genital skin-to-skin contact or by the virus traveling on hands, fingers, or sex toys. Since HPV can be spread by women who have sex with women, and because sex with a man could have occurred at some point in a woman's sexual history, all women, regardless of sexual preferences, lifestyle, or practices should have regular HPV screening with a Pap test.

Prevention

Gay and lesbian individuals can follow the same preventive measures as heterosexual individuals to avoid transmitting or contracting STDs. Overall risks for STDs can be lowered by limiting the number of sex partners one has and ideally having sex with only one person who is only having sex with them. Barrier methods remain the most effective way of preventing the transmission of STDs between partners. For men, the proper and consistent use of condoms can protect men from a majority of STDs. For women, dental dams provide a protective barrier. Dental dams are thin, square pieces of latex, rubber, or silicone that can be placed over the labia or the anus during oral-vaginal or oral-anal intercourse. Finger cots, additionally, are latex covers that can protect the fingers, and the vaginal mucous membranes, from transmitting microorganisms through skin-to-skin contact of the fingers or hands.

Gay and lesbian individuals, similar to heterosexual individuals, require individualized medical care from a health-care practitioner. The need for STD screening tests can be determined based upon a thorough review of a person's medical and sexual history. HIV testing should become a routine screening test during health maintenance visits. Lastly, both homosexual men and women can benefit from being vaccinated for HBV and HPV as appropriate.

10. Does being transgender affect my chances of contracting an STD?

"Transgender" is a term used to describe a person's gender identity or expression (i.e., masculine, feminine, and other) that is different from his or her sex (male or female) at birth. Being transgender itself does not impact a person's chances of contracting an STD. However, similar to any man or woman, the sexual behaviors or health factors of a transgender individual are what put them at greatest risk for contracting STDs. According to the CDC, transgender women, for example, have a very high chance of contracting HIV, a 49-times greater risk than the non-transgender population. Further, black/African American transgender individuals have the highest number of positive HIV test results in the United States, with 99 percent of all HIV positive transgender people being trans female. Similarly, HIV prevalence among transgender men is relatively low, but recent studies suggest that transgender MSM are at substantial risk for acquiring HIV. It is the risk factors, then, that predispose transgender people to contracting STDs.

There are many cultural, socioeconomic, and health-related factors that may contribute to the increased prevalence of STDs among transgender people. Sexual behaviors among transgender people vary, but the practice of unprotected anal receptive sex is a common trend reported in studies of the transgender community. Additionally, sex with multiple partners, exchanging sex for drugs or money, and prostitution, have all been implicated as sexual behaviors that increase the risk of STDs for the transgender community. Indeed, studies of transgender people reveal societal rejection and marginalization within society, with homelessness, poverty, and lack of access to sensitive, quality health care as contributing to the increased incidence of STDs within the transgender community.

Without adequate employment, health insurance, or health care, many transgender people have their signs and symptoms of STDs undiagnosed. Despite the increased incidence of HIV in the transgender community, studies demonstrate that transgender people are less likely to be maintained on antiretroviral therapy (ART), or achieve viral suppression. It is possible, then, for transgender people to transmit the microorganisms that cause STDs on to their sex partners through oral, vaginal, or anal sex.

Transgender people, therefore, are equally at risk for contracting and transmitting STDs. Risky sexual behaviors, then, are the common factor that put all individuals, regardless of gender identity or expression, at equal risk for STDs. Signs and symptoms of STDs will manifest in male or female genitalia, regardless of the individual's outward social expression of his or her gender. Prevention strategies, then, apply equally to transgender individuals. More research, however, is needed to determine how to best serve the transgender community and identify ways to accurately collect data pertinent to this community.

11. Can I still get pregnant in the future if I had an STD?

It is widely known that unprotected sex can lead to serious diseases, including STDs. However, what is a lesser-known fact is that STDs can also cause problems with an existing pregnancy and lead to fertility problems in the future. Each year, more women are discovering that they are unable to get pregnant because of an STD. Some women, further, do not know they have an STD until they struggle to become pregnant and seek a medical evaluation from a health-care practitioner. Many of the STDs experienced by women, additionally, may have been contracted years prior.

According to recent reports, an estimated 111 million new cases of curable STDs, and half of all new HIV infections, occur among young people. Many STDs, however, go unnoticed and untreated because there are often no symptoms of disease. STDs compromise fertility because, for women, the microorganisms that contribute to STDs invade and linger in the structures of the female upper genital tract. In men, though less common, the microorganisms invade and linger in the vas deferens in the scrotum that leads to scarring or obstruction. Left untreated, STDs, then, can lead to irreversible scarring of the fallopian tubes, which impairs a woman's ability to become pregnant, or block the outflow of sperm that is needed to unite with an ovum for fertilization to occur.

Not every STD will affect a woman's ability to become pregnant or carry a baby to full term, but several can. Similarly, specific STDs can impact the viability of male sperm. Specific STDs, and the issues they cause, include:

Herpes: The herpes virus itself does not directly affect a man or woman's ability to have a baby. However, during an outbreak of herpes lesions, couples are required to abstain from sex, thereby limiting the couple's chances of conceiving depending upon the duration of the outbreak or how frequently the outbreak occurs. If a woman experiences a herpes outbreak while in the later stages of pregnancy, it is recommended that a woman have a Cesarean birth as opposed to a vaginal birth to ensure the virus does not spread to the baby during delivery.

Chlamydia: The STD that is the largest threat to fertility is chlamydia. It is estimated that a million new cases of chlamydia are reported in the United States each year; a majority of women with chlamydia, however, are unaware they have the disease. Left untreated, chlamydia ascends into the female upper genital tract and typically invades the fallopian tubes. The inflammation that follows can leave scarring in the fallopian tubes, which blocks an ovum's transport for fertilization and implantation. Worse, the blocked fallopian tubes can halt the progress of a fertilized ovum directly, leaving the fertilized ovum to undergo its cellular changes and growth trapped inside the fallopian tube. Known as an ectopic pregnancy, the growing ovum undergoes improper cellular changes and grows in size rapidly. If left untreated, the fallopian tube can be further damaged, or ruptured, creating numerous medical complications for a woman, including permanent infertility.

Trichomoniasis: Untreated trichomoniasis causes inflammation of the fallopian tubes that can permanently scar, and block, the fallopian tubes. Similar to the effects of chlamydia, scarred or blocked fallopian tubes can impair a woman's ability to conceive.

Gonorrhea: Untreated gonorrhea results in damage to the cervix, or the opening of the uterus. The bleeding that often occurs after sex, coupled with yellow or bloody vaginal discharge, leads to inflammation in the pelvic area that hinders conception. Gonorrhea, like other STDs that invade the cervix, can weaken the cervix's integrity and, especially if a woman is pregnant, impair her ability to carry a baby to full term. Gonorrhea in men can invade the testicles and cause inflammation of the epididymis (called epididymitis) which hinders the production of sperm.

Since several STDs can impact both a man and woman's fertility, the need for preconception screening is essential to identify any preexisting conditions that could impact a couple's ability to conceive a baby, or a woman's ability to carry her baby to full term and have a vaginal delivery. Preconception screening, then, includes a thorough medical and sexual history review by a health-care practitioner, a complete physical examination, and a pelvic examination for women with a Pap test and other panel of screening tests for the presence of STDs.

12. Can an STD be transmitted to my baby if I get pregnant?

STDs can complicate pregnancy and may have serious consequences for both a woman and her developing baby. Some STDs can be passed to a baby by its mother during pregnancy, while other STDs have more impact on the pregnancy itself. Prenatal care, then, is essential for monitoring that a baby is growing and developing properly and that a mother remains free of illnesses or complications. Screening tests for STDs specifically occur in the first prenatal visits and may be repeated close to delivery. The CDC has established recommendations to health-care practitioners for screening pregnant women that include specimens to obtain during a pelvic examination and laboratory blood tests to order. The CDC, further, recommends treatment regimens where appropriate that are safe to take during pregnancy, and when to retest or rescreen women.

Specific STDs have varying impact on a developing baby or a pregnancy. The STDs include:

Bacterial vaginosis (BV): BV during pregnancy is associated with serious pregnancy complications including premature rupture of membranes that surround the baby in the uterus (i.e., a woman's water breaks too early or at a time when the baby is too small or premature if delivery follows), preterm or early labor, premature birth, or an infection of the membranes surrounding the baby (called chorioamnionitis) or the inner lining of the uterus itself (called endometritis). Women at high risk for preterm delivery should be screened for BV. There are no known direct effects, however, of BV on a developing baby.

Chlamydia: The most common bacterial STD in the United States, chlamydia can be contracted before or during pregnancy. Untreated chlamydia during pregnancy has been linked to preterm labor, premature rupture of membranes, and low birth weight babies. The newborn can become infected with chlamydia during delivery as the baby passes through the birth canal. Newborns exposed to chlamydia can develop serious eye or lung infections. Antibiotics, however, can be safely given to mothers while pregnant if chlamydia is diagnosed.

Gonorrhea: Similar to chlamydia, gonorrhea is a common bacterial STD in the United States. Untreated gonorrhea in pregnancy has been linked to miscarriages, premature birth, low birth weight babies, premature rupture of membranes, and chorioamnionitis. Gonorrhea can infect an infant during delivery as it passes through the birth canal, leading to serious eye infections. Because gonorrhea can cause problems in both the mother and her baby, it is important that the infection is treated properly. Antibiotics can safely be given to mothers while pregnant and follow-up testing is recommended to ensure the treatment was successful to cure the gonorrhea.

Hepatitis B: A mother can transmit the HBV to her baby during pregnancy. While the risk of an infected mother transmitting the HBV to her baby varies, depending on when she becomes pregnant, the greatest risk happens, however, when a mother becomes infected close to the time of delivery. Infected newborns, then, are at higher risk of becoming chronic HBV carriers themselves, with an increased risk of developing chronic liver disease or liver cancer later in life. However, vaccines are available for mothers prior to becoming pregnant to prevent against Hepatitis B, and treatment options, and vaccinations, are available for infants shortly after birth.

Hepatitis C: Hepatitis C virus (HCV) can be passed, like HBV, from an infected mother to her baby during pregnancy. The risk of a mother transmitting the HCV to her baby is higher if the mother is also infected with HIV. Infants born to Hepatitis C-infected mothers are typically small for their gestational age, premature, and have a low birth weight. Newborns with Hepatitis C, however, usually do not have symptoms and a majority will clear the infection without active medical treatment.

Herpes: The two distinct HSV types that can infect the human genital tract are HSV-1 and HSV-2. Most infections in the newborn are caused by HSV-2. Although transmission may occur during pregnancy and after delivery, the risk of transmission to the neonate from an infected mother is higher among women who acquire genital herpes near the time of delivery, and lower among women with recurrent herpes or who acquire the infection during the first half of pregnancy. HSV infection can have serious effects on newborns, especially if the mother's first outbreak occurred during the third trimester. Cesarean section is recommended, then, for all women in labor with active genital herpes lesions or early symptoms. Antiviral medications, however, do little to protect a baby while in utero from exposure to HSV.

HIV: The most common ways that HIV passes from mother to baby are during pregnancy, labor, delivery, or through breastfeeding. However, when HIV is diagnosed before or during pregnancy, and appropriate treatment and follow-up occur, the risk of mother-to-baby transmission is lowered.

Human papillomavirus: HPV are viruses that most commonly thrive in the lower genital tract, including the cervix, vagina, and external genitalia. Genital warts, if present, frequently increase in size and number during pregnancy. If a woman has genital warts during pregnancy, treatment may have to be postponed until after delivery. When large or too numerous, genital warts can complicate a vaginal delivery. A Cesarean birth may be recommended.

Syphilis: Syphilis can be transmitted to a baby by an infected mother during pregnancy. Syphilis has been linked to premature births, stillbirths, and, in some cases, infant death shortly after birth. Transmission of syphilis to a developing baby, further, can lead to a serious multisystem infection known as congenital syphilis. Congenital syphilis, additionally, are increasing in the United States. Antibiotic treatment for mothers is available to both treat syphilis and prevent transmission of the disease to a baby. Untreated syphilis in infants, if they survive, develops problems in multiple organs including the brain, eyes, heart, skin, teeth, or bones.

Trichomoniasis: Although most women will report no symptoms of trichomoniasis, pregnant women often report itching, irritation, unusual odor, discharge, and pain with sex or urination. Trichomoniasis during pregnancy has been linked to premature rupture of membranes, preterm birth, and low birth weight babies.

STDs during Pregnancy

Bacterial or protozoan STDs, such as chlamydia, gonorrhea, syphilis and trichomoniasis can all be treated and cured with antibiotics that are safe to take during pregnancy. Viral STDs, including genital herpes, Hepatitis B, and HIV cannot be cured. However, in some cases, viral STDs can be treated with antiviral medications or preventive measures to decrease the risk of passing a viral STD on to a baby.

Sexual activity can continue during pregnancy for many women. The most reliable way to avoid transmission of STDs to a baby or an uninfected partner, including during pregnancy, is to abstain from oral, vaginal, or anal sex during pregnancy. However, if sexual activity is going to occur, the proper and consistent use of condoms, including when pregnant, can greatly reduce the transmission of harmful microorganisms that cause STDs and, ultimately, the transmission of those harmful microorganisms to an unborn baby.

13. If neither one of us has an orgasm, can we still get an STD?

An orgasm does not have to occur for either sex partner to transmit an STD. An orgasm is a feeling of intense sexual pleasure that happens during sexual activity. Often called the "climax" or "coming/cumming," orgasm differs in experience and duration for men and women. Both men and women, however, can experience orgasm and both can share similar physiologic responses of a faster heartbeat, quicker, heavier breathing, and a sensation of pleasure. For women, foreplay causes blood to rush to the vagina and the clitoris. Blood continues to flow to the pelvic area as stimulation increases. The sensation of orgasm is usually coupled with a release of generalized muscle tension in the body, while the genital muscles in the pelvic floor contract (i.e., the uterus, vagina, and anus contract simultaneously). The recovery period between orgasms for women is brief; a woman may experience multiple orgasms if she continues to be stimulated. Women, unlike men, do not ejaculate body fluids with orgasms. Some women, however, report a clear fluid leaking or spurting from the glands close to the urethra (i.e., the Skene's glands) during intense sexual excitement or orgasm.

Men, in contrast, reach orgasm and a rhythmic series of muscle contractions within and around the penis and throughout the pelvis cause an ejaculation of semen and seminal fluid from the tip of the penis. Semen amounts vary, but large quantities of sperm can be contained in small amounts of semen. Men, unlike women, have only one orgasm at a time; a recovery phase follows each male orgasm where the penis and testicles shrink back to their normal size. Repeated sexual activity can continue, but penetration, and ejaculation, can only occur after the recovery phase is completed. The recovery phase for men can last a few minutes to several hours.

STDs require contact with infected body fluids or skin-to-skin contact for some specific diseases to be transmitted. It is possible, then, for an uninfected person to come in contact with infected body fluids without an orgasm occurring. Infected body fluids include those found in the mouth, penis, vagina, or rectum. Those fluids are present at all times and do not require sexual activity, or orgasm, to increase in amount, volume, or ability to cause an STD.

A male orgasm, however, can deposit copious amounts of semen into a vagina or rectum if unprotected sex occurs. In addition to the other infectious body fluids a person may come in contact with, semen is thick and can coat or cover the surfaces of the vagina or rectum, thereby increasing the possibility of a man transmitting an STD through semen to a partner, or a partner contracting an STD because of exposure to semen.

It is clear, then, that an orgasm does not need to occur for transmission of the microorganisms that cause STDs to happen. There are multiple ways to come in contact with infectious body fluids, including direct touching or skin-to-skin contact, that are equally as powerful at transmitting, or sharing, STDs. The proper and consistent use of condoms or other barrier methods, throughout all phases or stages of sexual activity, including foreplay to rigorous sexual intercourse, affords the best protection currently against transmitting, or contracting STDs.

14. If I had an STD in the past, will it show up on a physical exam or in a blood test later?

If a person had certain STDs in the past that were successfully treated, there are no long-lasting effects or evidence that the STD ever occurred.

With some STDs, follow-up testing, or retesting, is needed to determine if the treatment regimen was successful or if additional treatment is necessary. When successful, no evidence of the STD will be identified on repeat testing.

What can occur, however, is that a person can be exposed to, and infected with, and STD and never developed symptoms. A person may undergo testing for various reasons that are ordered by a health-care practitioner (e.g., preconception evaluation, routine GYN exam) and the presence of the STD is discovered. There is no way, however, to pinpoint when exposure or infection occurred, only that an STD is present.

Certain aspects of STDs can be detected on laboratory blood tests and possibly during a physical examination. What is important to differentiate is that only some STDs can be diagnosed through blood tests, but only if those specific blood tests are ordered by a health-care practitioner. A majority of the STDs requires either direct visualization or inspection with specimens of any discharge obtained and sent to a laboratory for analysis. Regular physical examinations, for example, a preemployment physical or sports physical, do not include a pelvic examination for women. Similarly, these physical examinations for men usually involve an inspection and palpation of the male genitalia but do not usually involve invasive probing or obtaining specimens.

In relation to the common STDs and their ability to be picked up or discovered by routine laboratory blood work or a physical examination, the following exists in regard to potential findings:

Chlamydia and gonorrhea: Both chlamydia and gonorrhea are caused by bacteria, which live in the urethra in men and the cervix or vagina in women. Chlamydia and gonorrhea may occur separately or both infections can occur simultaneously. It is possible for a person infected with both to have no symptoms. However, if there is noticeable discharge, a health-care practitioner may notice this during a physical examination and investigate further. Otherwise, there are usually no outward signs that either STD occurred, nor is there a blood test that would identify its presence.

Syphilis: Blood tests are available to determine the presence of syphilis. While not part of routine laboratory blood tests, certain professions (e.g., health-care workers) are required to be tested for syphilis prior to employment or working with sick people and those with compromised immunity.

Herpes: Active herpes infection where sores, lesions, or ulcers are present in or around the mouth, penis, or on the vagina or buttocks may be found during a routine physical examination. However, routine blood tests do not reveal the presence of HSV-1 or HSV-2; blood test for herpes can be expensive and often require a special order from a health-care practitioner.

HPV: Only a visible wart found on the genitals during a physical examination would signify that a person was infected with HPV at some point. Routine laboratory tests, however, will not detect the presence of HPV; even if a person was vaccinated against HPV, there is no routine laboratory blood test that determines immunity to the virus.

Hepatitis B: Similar to syphilis, there are blood tests available that test for the presence of HBV itself (HBV-Ag) or antibodies to it (HBV-Ab). Since there is widespread availability of the Hepatitis B vaccine, it is not uncommon to routinely check levels of immunity (i.e., the presence of antibodies) with blood tests during a routine physical examination. Further, for specific professions, such as health-care workers, routine screening is required as part of pre-employment physical examinations and periodically thereafter to evaluate ongoing immunity. However, unless a person is acutely ill with Hepatitis B, a physical examination alone will not detect the presence of the HBV.

HIV: Similar to other STDs, unless there are specific symptoms or signs of active disease, a physical examination will not detect the presence of HIV. There are blood tests for detecting HIV. However, HIV testing has requirements for pretesting counseling, follow-up and consenting procedures that vary state by state. A health-care practitioner, clinic, school, or employer cannot test a person for HIV randomly or without the person's consent. Like the other STDs, a positive blood test for HIV can only identify the presence of HIV and does not determine when the infection occurred.

Different Types of STDs

15. What is chlamydia?

One of the most discreet, yet the most common bacterial STD, is chlamydia. Men and women infected with chlamydia often are not aware that they even have chlamydia because, typically, there are no symptoms of an active infection. Since there are no symptoms that compel a person to seek treatment, there is an increased likelihood of repeatedly passing the chlamydia bacterium from partner to partner or to repeatedly exposing the same partner to the disease. According to the Centers for Disease Control (CDC), chlamydia is most common among young people, with almost two-thirds of new chlamydia infections among people aged 15–24. Further, it is estimated that 1 in 20 sexually active women aged 14 to 24 has chlamydia. Because chlamydia infection occurs so frequently and is without symptoms, screening for the disease has become a routine procedure during annual health examinations or during routine gynecological exams.

The microorganism that causes chlamydia is a bacterium known as *Chlamydia trachomatis* (or *C. trachomatis*). The bacterium is transmitted through sexual contact with the penis, vagina, mouth, or anus of an infected partner. Ejaculation of semen into the vagina, anus, or mouth does not need to occur in order to transmit chlamydia; the disease can be transmitted by external contact with genital-to-genital contact of an infected person (e.g., when the tip of the penis is rubbed across the vagina or its opening, or the rectum). Similarly, men engaging in homosexual sex can easily transmit the bacterium to another man through oral or anal sex. If untreated, chlamydia can also be spread from a mother to her baby during childbirth.

Signs and Symptoms

Initially, there are no outward signs that a person is infected with chlamydia (e.g., redness, rash, sores, or odors in the genital area). Typically, there are no symptoms experienced by people infected with the chlamydia bacterium; most people will remain without symptoms, especially women. If any symptoms were to develop, while not common, they may appear in as little as 5–10 days after being infected.

Men and women will exhibit different symptoms. For example, men may report pain or burning while urinating, pus or a watery-milky discharge or drainage from the tip or opening of the penis, swollen or tender testicles, or swelling of the anus or rectal opening. In contrast, women may experience abdominal pain or abnormal vaginal discharge. Additionally, women may also experience bleeding or spotting between menstrual periods, have a low grade fever (i.e., 99–100.6° Fahrenheit), painful sexual intercourse, pain or burning while urinating, or swelling inside the vagina, vaginal opening, or the rectum. A woman may notice an increased urge to urinate more frequently (and may often believe she has a urinary tract infection), or notice new vaginal bleeding or spotting after sexual intercourse. Less common, but possible, for women is the presence of a yellowish, foul-smelling, often itchy or irritating vaginal discharge.

Though not as common as infections in the genital areas, chlamydia can also infect the eyes or throat if either of these areas comes in contact with the chlamydia bacterium. For example, it is possible for the eyes to come in contact with the bacterium during oral sex or the eyes to be splashed with infected semen during male ejaculation. If the eyes are infected with chlamydia, redness, itching or discharge from the eye may occur that is often mistaken for, or mimics, the symptoms of "pink eye." Similarly, chlamydia can infect the mucous membranes of the throat during oral sex or with the swallowing of semen from an infected male partner. The most common symptom of a chlamydia infection in the throat is soreness or painful swallowing that is often confused with similar symptoms experienced with an upper respiratory tract infection or strep throat.

Diagnosis

Because infection with chlamydia is so common, routine screening is performed during annual health examinations for sexually active men and women. Fortunately, there are highly sensitive diagnostic tests that accurately identify chlamydia. For both men and women, cultures can be taken directly from the cervix within the vagina, or from the surface inside the penis, rectum, throat, or on the surface of the eyes. A small, soft, cotton-tipped probe is swabbed across the surface of the area in question and is sent off to a laboratory for analysis to identify the *C. trachomatis* bacterium. Depending on the laboratory, results may be available within 24 hours to 1 week. Similarly, a urine test has been developed that is reliable for screening for the presence of the chlamydia bacterium. A urine test is easier and convenient to obtain but is often used for routine screening or chlamydia. When any symptoms of chlamydia are present, or if a definitive diagnosis is needed, culture swabs of a potentially infected surface are the best method to obtain a diagnosis.

Treatment

Chlamydia is treatable and curable. Most physicians or other practitioners will often collect a specimen for diagnosis and implement treatment immediately as opposed to waiting for test results to come back. Additionally, because chlamydia and gonorrhea (another STD caused by a bacterium) often occur together, or one disease can mask the symptoms of the other, health-care practitioners will often treat someone for both diseases at the same time without waiting for cultures to confirm the diagnosis. Standard treatment for both chlamydia and gonorrhea is antibiotic pills that are taken orally. Regardless if someone is allergic to antibiotics, there are various regimens available that successfully eliminate chlamydia. In fact, one highly effective option is a single dose of antibiotic pills taken orally one time only.

Unlike other STDs, chlamydia, once diagnosed, requires all partners of the infected person to be treated as well. Even if sexual partners do not have any symptoms of an active chlamydia infection, they can still be active carriers of the disease. The likelihood, then, of a partner reinfecting someone who may have just completed treatment, infecting other sexual partners, or developing active infection themselves, is high. Depending on where one seeks treatment for chlamydia, some physicians or practitioners may provide a prescription for an infected person's partner without the need for an examination or testing. However, testing all partners of infected people properly, and prescribing the appropriate treatment individualized to each person, is ideal.

While one is being treated for chlamydia, one should abstain from sex and sexual activity for several days until symptoms subside or the antibiotic regimen is completed. Until all partners are treated, one should protect themselves from reinfection, or prevent the spread of infection to a partner, by using condoms.

Additional Considerations

With an individualized, prescribed antibiotic regimen, chlamydia can be reliably cured. Left untreated, however, long-term consequences can follow, especially for women more than men. Specifically, damage to the uterus or fallopian tubes is a real consequence of untreated chlamydia. Consequences, then, include the development of pelvic inflammatory disease (PID), a condition where the microorganisms that cause an STD to ascend up into the uterus and fallopian tubes causing widespread inflammation and pain. Additionally, there is an increased risk for ectopic pregnancy (i.e., a potentially life-threatening condition where a pregnancy develops in the fallopian tube instead of the uterus), chronic pelvic pain, or infertility.

Once treatment is completed, some physicians or practitioners may opt to retest infected people to verify that the treatment was successful. Follow-up typically occurs within 2–3 months where culture swabs, again, are taken from within the vagina, penis, or rectum to test for the presence of the chlamydia bacterium. If treatment was successful, repeat tests will be negative or fail to detect the presence of the chlamydia bacterium. Additional counseling and education is often provided at the follow-up visit to empower men and women with knowledge to prevent reinfection with chlamydia.

Prevention

Anyone who is sexually active with multiple partners or outside of a monogamous relationship, essentially, is at risk for contracting chlamydia. Additionally, anyone who has any symptoms of genital discharge, burning with urination, unusual sores or a rash is suspect for having been infected with chlamydia. For people showing any of those signs or symptoms, they should avoid all forms of sexual contact or use condoms until they have a full evaluation by a physician or health-care practitioner. Additionally, people who engage in specific at-risk behaviors such a having sex with new, or multiple, sex partners, or sex with a partner who is already infected with gonorrhea or other STDs, should seek more frequent screening and surveillance by a health-care practitioner. Further, women who have had chlamydia in the past, or who have recently completed treatment for the disease, and are anticipating pregnancy should consult with a health-care practitioner to receive a full evaluation and screening prior to becoming pregnant, along with additional follow-up and screening once pregnancy is confirmed.

16. What is gonorrhea?

Gonorrhea is another common bacterial sexually transmitted disease. According to the CDC, it is estimated that approximately 820,000 new gonorrheal infections occur in the United States each year. Similar to chlamydia, gonorrhea occurs most frequently among people aged 15–24 with men and women equally at risk for contracting the disease. Any sexually active person, however, can be infected with gonorrhea. In the United States currently, the highest reported rates of gonorrhea infections are among sexually active teens, young adults, and African Americans.

Gonorrhea is caused by a bacterial microorganism, *Neisseria gonorrhoeae* (*N. gonorrhoeae*). *N. gonorrhoeae* infects the mucous membranes, or inner lining and tissues, of the reproductive tract. For women, *N. gonorrhoeae* typically invades the cervix, uterus, fallopian tubes, or the urethra (the opening through which urine passes out of the body). In men, because the penis has only one opening that is used to pass both urine out of the body and ejaculate semen, *N. gonorrhoeae* typically will only infect the lining of the urethra. Both men and women, however, can also have *N. gonorrhoeae* infect the mucous membranes of the mouth, throat, and rectum, similar to chlamydia.

Gonorrhea is transmitted through sexual contact with the penis, mouth, or rectum of an infected partner. Similar to chlamydia, ejaculation does not have to occur for gonorrhea to be transmitted or acquired; the disease can be transmitted by external contact with the genitals of an infected person (e.g., when the tip of the penis of an infected man is rubbed across the vagina or its opening, or the rectum). Similarly, men engaging in homosexual sex can easily transmit the bacterium (*N. gonorrhoeae*) to another man through oral or anal sex.

Signs and Symptoms

Most men and women with gonorrhea have no symptoms and often do not know they have the disease at all. If symptoms are experienced, men and women differ in the symptoms they may experience. Men with gonorrhea typically experience a thick white, yellow, or green discharge from the tip of the penis that can appear anywhere from one day to two weeks after being exposed to the *N. gonorrhoeae* bacterium. Often men will experience burning or painful urination, along with intermittent itching at the tip of the penis. Men, further, may also notice dried white or yellow staining on the front of their underwear. Women, if they have symptoms at all, may often mistake them for a bladder infection or vaginal yeast infection. Women with gonorrhea may notice slight burning with urination or a milky white, slightly odorous vaginal discharge. Often there is itching or a burning sensation at the vaginal opening or within the vagina. Women may also notice irregular vaginal bleeding or spotting between periods.

Gonorrhea, like chlamydia, can infect the rectum or throat for both men and women. When there is an infection in the rectum, both men and women may notice increased drainage or loose, oil-like mucous from the rectum. Many report annoying itching and discomfort at the rectal opening, pain with prolonged sitting or walking, painful bowel movements, or noticeable blood on toilet paper with wiping following a bowel movement. Most times, however, gonorrheal infections of the rectum have no symptoms at all. Conversely, when gonorrhea infects the throat both men and women report, similar to chlamydia, persistent sore throat and painful swallowing that is often mistaken for strep throat or an upper respiratory tract infection.

Diagnosis

Similar to chlamydia, routine screening for gonorrhea is performed during annual health examinations for sexually active men and women, or anyone presenting for an evaluation by a health-care practitioner with any symptoms that suggest gonorrhea or another STD. Like chlamydia, there are highly sensitive diagnostic tests that accurately identify gonorrhea. Some tests, in fact, can detect the presence of both gonorrhea and chlamydia at the same time with one single swab or culture. For both men and women, cultures taken from the genital areas (i.e., the penis, vagina, or rectum) are the most accurate for diagnosing gonorrhea. A urine test, also, is available, primarily for men, which is useful for diagnosing the presence of gonorrhea. Swabbing the inner surfaces of the penile opening, and a few inches inside the penis, with a small, cotton-tipped swab that is analyzed in a laboratory to identify the presence of the *N. gonorrhoeae* bacterium remains the best, most effective way of diagnosing gonorrhea in men. For women, a gynecologic examination where swabs taken from the cervix or vagina can be obtained and then examined in a laboratory for analysis to identify the presence of the *N. gonorrhoeae* bacterium remains the gold standard for diagnosing the presence of gonorrhea.

Treatment

Like chlamydia, physicians or other health-care practitioners will often not wait for cultures to be resulted before beginning someone on treatment. If the symptoms a person has, plus his or her sexual patterns or history, raises suspicion for gonorrhea, chlamydia, or both, treatment is typically started right away while awaiting the culture results. Fortunately, like chlamydia, gonorrhea is curable with the proper antibiotic regimen.

Presently, the CDC recommends using two different kinds of antibiotic pills to treat gonorrhea (as opposed to only one antibiotic that is used for treating chlamydia). There are various combinations of oral antibiotics for health-care practitioners to prescribe; even for people who are allergic to antibiotics, there are multiple alternative drugs, and combinations of drugs, that can be used to cure gonorrhea.

Like chlamydia, partners of people diagnosed with gonorrhea will need to be treated also. Typically, all sexual partners, regardless of length or type of contact, who the infected person has had contact with in the past 60 days before the onset of symptoms or diagnosis, should be treated. Even if the sexual partners have no symptoms, the likelihood of someone reinfecting their current partner, or infecting someone else, is high. Depending on where one seeks health care, some health-care practitioners may provide a prescription for antibiotics for someone's partner without the need for an examination or testing by the health-care practitioner. However, similar to chlamydia, testing all partners properly, and prescribing the appropriate treatment individualized to each person, is ideal. Further, since gonorrhea infection often has no symptoms, proper evaluation and treatment of all sexual partners helps minimize some of the serious complications of untreated, or improperly treated, gonorrhea.

Additional Considerations

Like chlamydia, untreated gonorrhea can lead to a multitude of complications for the person infected with gonorrhea, for women more so than men. Untreated gonorrhea typically spreads to the uterus and fallopian tubes and leads to a condition call PID. PID is a condition where the microorganisms that cause an STD ascend up into the uterus and fallopian tubes causing widespread inflammation and pain. With PID caused by gonorrhea, then, there is a higher incidence of scarring of the fallopian tubes that leads to a greater chance of an ectopic pregnancy (a potentially life-threatening condition where a pregnancy develops in the fallopian tube instead of the uterus) or possible infertility. For men, untreated gonorrhea often leads to permanent infertility.

While one is being treated for gonorrhea, one should abstain from sex and sexual activity for several days until the symptoms subside or the antibiotic regimen is completed. It is still possible to transmit gonorrhea to a partner while undergoing treatment. Therefore, until all treatment is completed for the person infected and his or her partners are completed, one should protect themselves from reinfection, or prevent the spread of gonorrhea to a partner, by using condoms. Similarly, if the person infected is undergoing treatment and notices no improvement in symptoms, or is having an adverse reaction to the antibiotic regimen, it is necessary to contact the prescribing health-care practitioner to reevaluate all symptoms and potentially alter the treatment plan.

Once treatment is completed, some practitioners may opt to retest people that were diagnosed with gonorrhea to verify that the treatment was successful. Follow-up typically occurs within 2–3 months where swabs, or specimens, are taken again from within the vagina, penis, or rectum and tested to identify the presence of the *N. gonorrhoeae* bacterium. If successful, the test will be negative, or not detect the presence of the *N. gonorrhoeae* bacterium. Additional counseling is often provided at the follow-up visit to empower men and women with knowledge to prevent reinfection with gonorrhea.

Prevention

Anyone who is sexually active with multiple partners or outside of a monogamous relationship, essentially, is at risk for contracting gonorrhea. Additionally, anyone who has any symptoms of genital discharge, burning with urination, unusual sores or a rash is suspect for having been infected with gonorrhea. For people showing any of those signs or symptoms, they should avoid all forms of sexual contact or use condoms until they have a full evaluation by a physician or health-care practitioner. Additionally, people who engage in specific at-risk behaviors such as having sex with new, or multiple, sex partners, or sex with a partner who is already infected with gonorrhea or other STDs, should seek more frequent screening and surveillance by a health-care practitioner. Further, women who have had gonorrhea in the past, or who have recently completed treatment for the disease, and are anticipating pregnancy should consult with a health-care practitioner to receive a full evaluation and screening prior to becoming pregnant, along with additional follow-up and screening once pregnancy is confirmed.

17. What is trichomoniasis?

Trichomoniasis (or "trich") is the most prevalent, nonviral STD in the United States, affecting 3.7 million people according to the CDC. Trichomoniasis is caused by a protozoan called *Trichomonas vaginalis*, or *T. vaginalis*. Like many other STDs, men and women who have the protozoan often cannot tell they are infected. Only 30 percent of those infected develop any symptoms, with infection in women more common than men. Older women are more likely than younger women to have been infected.

The protozoan that causes trichomoniasis is passed from an infected person to an uninfected person during sexual activity. During sex, the protozoan is usually transmitted from the penis to the vagina or from the vagina to the penis. Unlike other STDs, trichomoniasis does not live on skin surfaces nor is it passed by casual contact. It requires the mucous membranes of the penis or the vagina to survive and flourish. Therefore, the most commonly infected body parts of women include those in the lower genital tract such as the urethra, the vaginal opening, and the vagina. In men, the protozoan thrives on the inner lining of the penis.

Signs and Symptoms

About 70 percent of people infected with *T. vaginalis* have no signs or symptoms of the disease. Even without symptoms, an infected person is capable of passing the protozoan on to an uninfected person. When symptoms of trichomoniasis do occur, they range from a mild irritation in the genital area to severe inflammation. The problem with trichomoniasis is that symptoms, if any, may come and go, or not appear, until 5 to 28 days (or later) after a person is infected. Symptoms, then, vary between men and women. Men with trichomoniasis may feel itching, burning, or irritation inside the penis that worsens after urinating or ejaculating semen. Additionally, men may notice a cloudy or white to gray, thick, slightly malodorous discharge from the tip of the penis that stains or leaves a residue on the inside front of their underwear. Women, in contrast, often report itching or burning in the genital areas that progress to irritation and soreness. There is typically pain, burning, or stinging at the urinary opening with urination. A thin, sticky, slightly fishy or malodorous, clear or white or pale yellow-to-light green discharge from the vagina may be present. The odor of trichomoniasis is unique and for most women unlike any other they may have experienced. The odor tends to worsen as the day progresses and does not diminish or disappear with douching or showering. Because the vagina or urethra in a woman are most often affected, sexual activity becomes more painful as the infection progresses. For many women, the vaginal redness, soreness, and itching are intensified by sex so they are likely to avoid sex as often as possible.

Because trichomoniasis causes inflammation of the lower genital tract, the skin and mucous membranes in those areas are more susceptible to injury such as abrasions or slight tearing that can serve as a portal of entry for other microorganisms, including HIV. Additionally, with the protozoan flourishing with the mucous membranes of the penis, the vagina, or both, it is easy to repeatedly pass the protozoan from partner to partner during unprotected sex. Further, women with trichomoniasis who become pregnant are more likely to develop the infection in the cervix. Cervical trichomoniasis during pregnancy, then, weakens the integrity of the cervical tissue and could potentially lead to preterm labor and the delivery of a premature or low birth weight baby.

Diagnosis

Diagnosing trichomoniasis requires a thorough evaluation by a health-care practitioner. Symptoms alone are not sufficient to diagnose trichomoniasis because the symptoms are similar to many of the other STDs. Trichomoniasis is harder to diagnose in men than in women. However, the characteristic odor of the vaginal discharge in women is often the first clue for a health-care practitioner to pursue a diagnosis of trichomoniasis.

Trichomoniasis is only diagnosed through laboratory testing. The gold standard is to take a sample of the vaginal fluid or from the inner lining of the penis, allowing it to grow in a culture medium, then examining it under a microscope to identify *T. vaginalis*. Currently, there are newer, faster tests such a rapid antigen tests and nucleic acid amplification that speed up the process of identifying the protozoan and expediting treatment.

Treatment

Trichomoniasis is curable. Often a single dose of prescription antibiotic medication such as metronidazole, or Flagyl, taken by mouth is sufficient to kill the protozoan and eliminate the infection. The treatment is safe for most people, including pregnant women. There are no over-the-counter medications available to treat trichomoniasis. Similarly, there are no soaps or douches that will eliminate trichomoniasis; prescription antibiotic medication is the only successful available treatment.

Despite successful treatment, many people who have been treated for trichomoniasis get it again. All sex partners, then, need to be treated also, regardless if symptoms are present. Since one in five people, according to the CDC, get reinfected with trichomoniasis within three months after treatment, it is recommended that infected persons avoid sexual activity for at least a week, or until symptoms, if any, subside. If symptoms do not subside, or recur, another evaluation by a health-care practitioner is required. Often treatment is repeated with each episode of trichomoniasis.

Additional Considerations

People infected with trichomoniasis are not required to notify partners of their diagnosis. However, treating partners is an important step in eliminating the disease and minimizing its spread. Treatment regimens have been simplified to a one-time oral dose of antibiotics. Side effects of the treatment are few and treatment is typically, successful. There is no way to tell if someone has, or is being treated for, trichomoniasis. The characteristic malodorous discharge in women is typically a late sign and most people outside of health care cannot readily detect the odor of trichomoniasis. Additionally, honest, open dialogue with a health-care practitioner will ensure adequate screening and testing is performed during a health visit.

Prevention

Since sexual activity is how trichomoniasis is transmitted from an infected person to an uninfected person, the proper and consistent use of condoms is the best way to reduce the risk of getting, or spreading, trichomoniasis. Trichomoniasis is spread when there is direct contact between mucous membranes and either semen or vaginal fluid. Therefore, other forms of birth control, including oral contraceptive pills, spermicides, diaphragms, or an intrauterine device are powerless to prevent trichomoniasis from occurring. Additionally, trichomoniasis is one of the STDs that can infect healthy people; no nutritional or exercise regimen can fortify a body enough to prevent trichomoniasis.

18. What are genital herpes?

Genital herpes is one of the STDs that, once contracted, will never completely disappear. While it can be controlled with various medications, a person with genital herpes is susceptible to repeated outbreaks throughout their lives. What makes genital herpes different than most other STDs is the fact that the microorganism that causes genital herpes is a virus as opposed to a bacterium or protozoan that is common with many of the other STDs. Bacteria, protozoans, or many other microorganisms can be cured with antibiotics; antibiotics, however, do not kill or cure viruses. Since there is no antibiotic or treatment to kill off the virus that causes genital herpes, the virus will remain in an infected person's body forever. After the initial outbreak of genital herpes, then, the symptoms subside and the virus then lies dormant in the infected person's body. What is concerning about genital herpes is that once the virus "wakes up" and begins to cause another flare-up or outbreak, that virus is contagious and can be easily transmitted through sexual activity days before the infected person ever begins to notice any symptoms. The focus with genital herpes, then, is recognizing the signs and symptoms early enough to begin anti-viral medication that will lessen the duration of the outbreak or flare-up, along with learning and controlling the various triggers that lead to an outbreak.

The word "herpes" has become a universal umbrella term to cover both genital herpes and herpes that infects other parts of the body. Though similar in certain aspects, the type of virus determines the type and location of a herpes outbreak. Oral herpes is caused by a form of the herpes virus call herpes simplex virus-type 1 (HSV-1). It is a unique strain of virus that infects the cells located in and around the mouth and face. With an outbreak of HSV-1, people experience a classic "cold sore," typically on the lips. The lesion can begin as a simple pimple or a break in the skin of the lips that progress to a painful, often fluid-filled blister that can linger for several days. Sometimes the lesions are within the mouth along the surface of the gum line or on the tongue itself. With HSV-1, oral-to-oral contact such as through kissing or sharing of lip balms or lipsticks easily transmits the virus from one person to another. Typically, like most viruses, HSV-1 is transmitted to another person long before the infected person who passed on the virus has any signs or symptoms of an impending outbreak.

Genital herpes, in contrast, is caused by another unique virus, herpes simplex virus-type 2. This virus has an affinity for the cells in and around the genital tract, especially the moist surfaces at the opening of the vagina, the opening at the tip of the penis, or around the rectum. Although the ulcer or blister that erupts is similar to those of oral herpes, the lesions in the genital tract are irritated more often since they come in contact with underwear, a stream or urine, menstrual bleeding, or feces from a bowel movement. Additionally, prolonged sitting or walking can cause further friction on a genital herpes lesion that contributes to additional pain and discomfort. The HSV-2 virus, like HSV-1, can lie dormant within an infected person for any length of time and, therefore, be transmitted easily to another person through vaginal or anal sex.

It is important to note that both HSV-1 and HSV-2 are not isolated to specific areas of the body. For example, a person with HSV-1 can transmit that virus to someone else through oral sex. A lesion in the genital tract could erupt, then, that is caused by HSV-1. Similarly, it is possible for an oral herpes lesion to erupt because of being infected by HSV-2. Though the recurrence rate of both is typically low when the atypical virus is the cause, transmission of the virus and the symptoms or duration of the outbreak remains the same.

Like many of the other STDs, the incidence of genital herpes is on the rise. What is more startling, genital herpes is becoming one of the most common STDs in women. Indeed, genital herpes is more easily transmitted from men to women than from women to men. What continues to complicate the avoidance of becoming infected with genital herpes is the fact that the HSV-2 virus is active and easy to transmit to another person days before any symptoms of an outbreak or flare-up are noticed by an infected person.

Genital herpes, then, is transmitted when a sex partner comes in contact with lesions that are in or on mucosal surfaces, such as those on the inside of the vagina. Additionally, genital or oral secretions or fluids can contain the HSV-2 virus. HSV-2 can be shed from skin surfaces that look completely normal; one does not need the presence of a lesion or obvious sore to shed the virus or be contagious. Often the infected person has no signs that they are infected or that an outbreak or flare-up may occur in several days. Having unprotected (i.e., without a condom) vaginal or anal sex, then, puts someone at risk for contracting genital herpes. Shedding, and possibly transmitting, the HSV-2 virus, further, can occur at any time over an infected person's life span, and an active infection or a repeated outbreak or flare-up does not need to occur for one to pass on the HSV-2 virus.

Signs and Symptoms

Most people will not know they have contracted genital herpes until an outbreak occurs; the average incubation period after exposure can range anywhere from 2–12 days. If symptoms appear, a person typically notices one or more vesicles (small, fluid-filled bumps that resemble clear pimples) on or around the penis, vagina, rectum, or the mouth. The vesicles grow and eventually break open or pop, leaving a painful ulcer or crater that can take two to four weeks to completely heal.

The initial outbreak of genital herpes is usually the longest, with most recurrent outbreaks taking less time to completely heal. During an initial infection or a recurrent outbreak, an infected person may also notice increased fatigue, muscle aches, fever, headache, or swollen lymph glands. Typically, as people experience recurrent outbreaks or flare-ups, they often recognize symptoms of an impending outbreak and report tingling or mild burning at a specific area where a vesicle is due to appear, or report pain in the legs, vagina, or buttocks days prior to a new lesion erupting.

Diagnosis

The pain and discomfort associated with genital herpes lesions are often what drives people to seek treatment. Because genital herpes lesions erupt close to, or within, the opening of the penis, vagina, or the rectum, the pain, burning or discomfort is often magnified and troublesome. A health-care practitioner will take a full health history and perform a physical examination of the affected area. While most genital herpes lesions have unique characteristics that can make them readily identifiable, some lesions could be indicative of other conditions. To help secure the diagnosis of genital herpes, the health-care practitioner will swab an active genital lesion with a cotton-tipped applicator and send the specimen as a viral culture to a laboratory to be examined and identified under a microscope for the presence of HSV-1 or 2. However, the older a lesion is, or the more it has healed, can limit the adequacy of the viral culture. Newer lesions, closer to the time of eruption, then, yield the best results. Additionally, blood tests are available to assist with diagnosing genital herpes, but the viral culture taken from an active lesion is preferred.

Treatment

There is no cure for herpes. There are no over-the-counter medications one can purchase, nor are the current topical medications available for cold sores indicated for, or effective against, genital herpes lesions. There is, however, antiviral medication that can shorten the duration of a genital herpes outbreak or prevent a future outbreak or flare-up from occurring. Several antiviral medications are available by prescription from a health-care practitioner that range in price from very affordable to expensive. Further, different antiviral drugs come with varying dosing regimens and schedule for when to take the medication. A health-care practitioner can customize a treatment plan depending on a person's specific needs.

Despite starting antiviral medication, a person remains capable of transmitting the virus. If outbreaks become more frequent, antiviral medication can be prescribed on a daily basis (called "suppressive therapy"). Suppressive therapy is aimed at minimizing the number, and severity, of outbreaks for the person infected with HSV-2. What suppressive therapy does not do is prevent an infected person from transmitting genital herpes to a sex partner. Sexual activity can be resumed, then, once the genital herpes lesion has healed and sexual contact is no longer painful. Condom use, however, is currently the best way to prevent transmission of genital herpes.

Additional Considerations

Genital herpes, and the ulcers or lesions that develop because of it, can pose significant issues or complications for certain groups of infected people. For example, people with HIV infection and weakened immune systems can become particularly ill from a genital herpes outbreak and are at increased risk of the ulcers or lesions becoming infected. Depending on the location of the lesion or ulcer, especially near the rectum, the area is prone to becoming infected and therefore takes longer to heal, leading to further pain and discomfort. People with genital herpes may touch the lesion or ulcer, thereby introducing bacteria into the area and potentially causing a secondary infection of the lesion and the surrounding tissue. It is also possible for a lesion to develop outside the genital area if a person touches the lesion or ulcer then touches other parts of his or her body such as the eyes or other skin surfaces.

Genital herpes is a particular concern for women who are pregnant or considering becoming pregnant. Herpes infections can be passed from mother to baby during pregnancy, childbirth, or immediately in the newborn period that can result in a potentially fatal neonatal herpes infection. If a woman contracts genital herpes for the first time during pregnancy, the risk of her transmitting herpes to her unborn baby are higher than if she were to experience a recurrent outbreak during pregnancy. Avoiding herpes in pregnancy, then, is important. Women are counseled to avoid intercourse and sexual activity during the third trimester of pregnancy with partners who are known to have, or suspected of having, genital herpes. Additionally, some women with a history of genital herpes may be offered to start a regimen of antiviral medications weeks prior to delivery. Once labor begins, however, women are carefully examined for the presence of genital herpes lesions to avoid transmitting a herpes infection to the baby during delivery as it passes through the birth canal. However, if the absence of lesions cannot be completely confirmed, women are often advised to avoid a vaginal birth; a Cesarean birth is recommended.

Prevention

There is no universal screening test for genital herpes. Further, there are no obvious ways for a person to know an actual or potential sex partner has genital herpes or is capable of transmitting the herpes virus. Therefore, the only way currently to avoid the risk of transmitting or contracting genital herpes is to abstain from sexual activity. Since complete abstinence from sexual activity is often not a viable option in today's society, the correct and consistent use of condoms, then, provides the only alternative to prevent transmitting or contracting genital herpes.

A person infected with genital herpes learns what triggers recurrent outbreaks of the infection. Specific environmental, physical, and psychological events can weaken one's immune system and produce a recurrent outbreak. For example, stress has been identified as a leading contributor to a recurrent outbreak. Stress, then, can take many forms including work-related stress, physical stress from being ill, or emotional stress from a major life event like a death of a family member or changing jobs, or day-to-day stress from trying to balance the demands of career, relationships, and other responsibilities. Lack of sleep and exercise, a poor diet, increased alcohol consumption, smoking, or drug use can also weaken one's immune system and predispose a person infected with genital herpes to a recurrent outbreak. As a person infected with genital herpes learns to navigate his or her disease, he or she can more readily identify situations that make him or her prone to a recurrent outbreak and therefore implement antiviral therapy sooner to minimize the severity of the outbreak or seek medical attention earlier to minimize the duration of the event.

A person infected with genital herpes carries a stigma related to the disease for life. A person with genital herpes, further, needs to admit to an actual or potential sex partner that he or she has the disease, while his or her sex partner has to weigh whether a relationship or sexual activity with the infected person is worth the risk of potentially contracting a lifelong disease. Having genital herpes, then, can be isolating and lead one to withdraw from meaningful relationships. However, with proper self-care, safe-sex practices, and attention to triggers that could lead to recurrent outbreaks, a person with genital herpes can still enjoy significant relationships with sex partners. Educating actual and potential partners, then, on the importance of correct and consistent use of condoms coupled with frank discussions about symptoms and occurrence of outbreaks can help minimize the stigma of the disease and promote worthwhile intimate relationships with partners.

19. What are genital warts?

Genital warts are a common STD that is typically an infection of the skin in and around the genital area (i.e., the penis, vagina, or rectum). Also called venereal warts or condylomata acuminata, these unsightly, often painful clusters of skin are caused by the human papillomavirus, or HPV. Since genital warts are caused by a virus, genital warts can never be cured. Managing the size and growth of the warts, however, is possible.

There are various strains of HPV, but only some are capable of causing genital warts. The strains of HPV that do cause genital warts (i.e., HPV 6 and HPV 11), however, are highly contagious and are passed easily from person to person with sexual contact. Genital warts themselves are also highly contagious. Unlike other STDs, HPV does not require breaks in the skin or mucous membranes to be transmitted. Skin-to-skin contact, then, is sufficient to transmit the disease from person to person. Because the HPV strains that lead to the development of genital warts are so contagious and capable of causing disease in most noninfected people who come in contact with it, an estimated 60 percent of people who come in contact with HPV during sexual activity will develop the disease. Genital warts, further, affect both men and women, but women are affected more and are more vulnerable to complications of the disease. More startling is the recent findings that among younger women aged 14 to 19, many were found to be carrying multiple strains of HPV believed to be due to younger women initiating sexual activity at early ages with multiple sex partners. Left untreated, genital warts can ultimately lead to the development of lethal cancers of the vagina, cervix, or uterus.

Once a person comes in contact with HPV, symptoms may develop within three months following the initial contact. In some cases, however, a person may have no obvious symptoms for several years. Regardless if symptoms are present, a person, once infected with HPV, can easily transmit the virus to sex partners.

Signs and Symptoms

Genital warts may not be visible to the human eye initially and may require evaluation by a health-care practitioner using special magnifiers.

Genital warts are not the same as warts that appear, for example, on the hands or other parts of the body. Genital warts, then, are often very small and usually the same tone and color of the skin or slightly darker. The top of the wart is often smooth but may be slightly bumpy to touch. There may be only one wart but often they appear in clusters. The clusters continue to grow and resemble cauliflower or mushroom bunches. They may be completely adhered to the skin or grow on a stalk. The larger they grow, the more tender they become or painful to the touch, especially when irritated by clothing. The skin covering the wart is thin and can easily bleed if scratched, such as when wiping after a bowel movement or drying with a towel. As the clusters grow, they become increasingly unsightly and can surround the urinary, vaginal, or rectal openings.

At the onset, men and women with genital warts often experience a burning sensation in the area where the wart is going to erupt or where it has erupted and is too small to see with the naked eye, or unable to be seen readily because it is inside the vagina or rectum. The area might be tender to touch or be aggravated when urine, menstrual flow, or bowel movements pass over the area. Itching is also a common complaint but scratching the area fails to relieve the itching and often makes the discomfort worse. Women may notice a mucous-like, or clear, vaginal discharge. Both men and women may complain of a tan to light brown discharge from the rectum if the warts are located in the rectal area.

Women often have warts that grow inside the vagina or rectum or along the outside skin of the vagina (called the labia majora). Sometimes the lesions grow internally and can be found on the cervix during a pelvic examination. Men, in contrast, often find warts along the shaft, or at the base, of the penis. Additionally, men often notice warts, or clusters of warts, on the scrotum, inside or around the anus, or along the inner thighs. Both men and women can experience warts orally on the lips, tongue, or inside the throat.

Diagnosis

The first step to diagnosing genital warts is to have a complete health and physical examination completed by a health-care practitioner. The genital areas will be examined closely, often with a light or magnifier to make inspecting the areas easier. For women, a pelvic examination is often included so the health-care practitioner can see the cervix and inner walls of the vagina. During the pelvic examination, a Pap test of the cervix is also obtained. The Pap test is a gentle swabbing, brushing, or scraping of the cervix to obtain cells from its surface. Aside from being able to detect the presence of HPV, the Pap test may also identify changes to the other cells or precancerous changes to the cervix that would warrant further evaluation or more frequent screening. For visible lesions, the health-care practitioner is able to swab the area and obtain a viral culture to diagnose the presence, and specific strain of, HPV. If a woman is pregnant, it is imperative to have a full examination by a health-care practitioner. HPV is transmissible to a baby from its mother during pregnancy. Therefore, proper diagnosis, and treatment, is essential prior to becoming pregnant or immediately after a woman discovers she is pregnant.

Treatment

Only visible warts can be treated. The type of treatment depends upon the location of the warts, how many warts there are, and what the warts look like. Treatment, then, is aimed at getting rid of the visible warts and lowering the amount of virus present. While there are several types of treatment available, such as medicated creams, freezing with liquid nitrogen, burning the warts off with electrocautery, surgical removal or removal with a laser, successful treatment does not guarantee the warts will not recur. Additionally, a combination of treatments is often the most effective. At present, there is no over-the-counter treatment one can buy to treat genital warts. Further, wart remover creams, gels, or pads that one would purchase over the counter and use on the hands or other parts of the body do not work on genital warts and should not be used. While genital warts will eventually go away if untreated, they tend to enlarge and become increasingly ugly or distressing to look at. Treating the warts, then, greatly reduces the risk of passing them on to another person and speeds the healing of the warts. Effective treatment, then, requires adhering to the prescribed treatment regimen and following-up with one's health-care practitioner as indicated.

Topical medicated creams are the most widely used treatment for genital warts. A medicated cream or liquid, available by prescription only, is applied directly onto the warts a few days each week. A person can apply these themselves at home. Over time, the warts begin to dry and shrink. Initially, the warts will become sore and flaky-appearing until healing begins. It is important to use the topical medication correctly. Care should be taken to wash your hands thoroughly before and after applying the cream, and use only the prescribed amount of cream applied only to the warts themselves. Using more medicated cream, or applying it to other places, does not speed the healing or removal of the warts or prevent new warts from forming. Treatment with topical medicated creams or liquids can take several weeks to complete.

Cryotherapy is another option for removing genital warts. Using liquid nitrogen spray, a health-care practitioner focuses a targeted blast from a specialized aerosol can or container to provide a direct application of liquid nitrogen to the wart. The liquid nitrogen freezes the skin and surface tissues of the wart and a blister forms. As the blister heals, the lesion, essentially, slides off, allowing new skin to grow where the wart was. While successful, repeated treatments spaced out over several intervals are often needed to fully remove the wart.

In contrast to using liquid nitrogen, a health-care practitioner can also use electric current to essentially burn, or fry off, genital warts. A local anesthetic is often used to numb the area prior to the treatment. Once the area is numb, an electrocautery is used that delivers an electric current which, in turn, produces heat that burns off the wart. Because the electrocautery produces heat, the tiny blood vessels that are at the base of, or part of, the wart are sealed shut in the burning process so bleeding, swelling, and bruising are minimized. While one treatment can be effective, additional treatments may be necessary to remove the wart.

Similar to electrocautery, lasers can also be used to remove genital warts. Instead of heat caused by an electric current, lasers create heat to burn off and remove genital warts by an intense beam of light. Like electrocautery, a local anesthetic is used to numb the area prior to using a laser. Protective eyewear is needed during the procedure for both the person being treated and the health-care practitioner. Unlike electrocautery, one treatment with laser can potentially remove genital warts effectively.

Surgical removal of genital warts remains a definitive option for treatment. With surgery, the warts, and the tissue that surround it, are cut out and the remaining edges of the tissues brought together with stitches. The surgical wound, then, heals like any other wound. Surgical removal requires local anesthetics to numb the area fully, or sometimes additional sedating medications to keep the person, or patient, comfortable and calm during the procedure. After the procedure, the person has to care for the surgical wound and take precautions to prevent an infection in the surgical wound. Healing of the wound depends on the health of the person and may take several weeks. Sexual activity is discouraged and should be avoided until the surgical wound is healed.

Prevention

The only definitive way to avoid genital warts is by not engaging in sexual activity at all (i.e., abstinence). Since abstinence is not a common or preferred option in modern times, barrier methods such as condoms help lower the risk of spreading HPV. Condoms, however, only cover a specific surface area of the penis or vagina. HPV is spread from skin-to-skin contact, so the genital region can still come in contact with HPV from touching the thighs, scrotum, or other genital skin of an infected person. With genital warts, further, most people often are unaware that they are infected and fail to use condoms properly and consistently to minimize any potential transmission of HPV.

Strains of HPV have been implicated in causing changes to a woman's cervix that could lead to cervical cancer. Because those changes are subtle and can occur over time, coupled with women and young girls initiating sexual activity at earlier ages with multiple partners over time, a vaccine was developed that could help protect women. Specifically, girls immunized at a young age are potentially protected from lethal cancers later in life. By vaccinating girls and boys between the ages of 9 to 26, it is hoped that protection against HPV will begin before the onset of sexual activity and remain with them through adulthood. In contrast, receiving the vaccine later in adulthood has demonstrated little to no efficacy against cervical cancers or genital warts. The HPV vaccine (known as Cervarix, Gardasil, and now Gardasil-9) not only protects against the various strains of HPV that cause cervical cancers but also protects against strains of HPV that cause 90 percent of genital warts. The vaccine, administered as a series of three injections spaced out over a six-month period, is not without controversy. While scientific evidence continues to demonstrate the efficacy of the vaccine, parents are reluctant to vaccinate their children in anticipation of a sexually transmitted disease or cancer that they may or may not get. Pediatricians, further, are divided among their professional organizations; opinions about whether or not to vaccinate are inconsistent. Despite the controversies surrounding the HPV vaccine, the scientific data regarding the HPV vaccine is compelling and encouraging regarding cervical cancers and genital warts. Careful analysis, then, of the risks and benefits of the vaccine should be explored and weighed by parents and health-care practitioners alike.

20. What is syphilis?

Syphilis is another STD that, once detected, can be successfully treated without the threat of long-term complications or consequence. However, if syphilis is not treated, or treated improperly, serious medical complications can follow. What makes treating syphilis properly a public health priority is that syphilis is one of the STDs that is easy to transmit to a sex partner or even to a baby during pregnancy. While several treatment regimens exist to cure syphilis, like many of the other STDs the signs and symptoms of syphilis are subtle and can often be overlooked or ignored.

Syphilis is caused by a bacterium, *Treponema pallidum* (or *T. pallidum*) that enters the body through any minute break in the skin or the mucous membranes of the genital area of the mouth. Once a person has come in contact with the bacterium, a chancre, or painless blister, sore or ulcer can develop, typically in the genital areas such as the penis, vagina, or rectum. Chancres can vary in size and length; some are tiny and can resemble a small paper cut, while others look like a tiny pimple. Chancres can be any size and shape but are most commonly circular, pink-to-red in color, and may have a small scab or crusting on top. The area surrounding the chancre may be reddened or a darker shade of pink. Some chancres ooze a scant amount of clear fluid, or may burn and itch when they come in contact with, or irritated by clothing, perspiration, or drops of urine. For a man, it is easier to examine his penis and identify a chancre. Women, however, often have a difficult time finding a chancre because they can be hidden within the vagina itself, around the urinary opening, or too tiny to see along the walls or skin of the vaginal opening. Similarly, anal chancres can be just as elusive and require a detailed examination in order to identify them properly. Chancres, at times, can also appear in or around the mouth.

While some people may have symptoms such as itching, burning, or pain when a chancre develops, many people have no symptoms or complaints during the first days that the chancre is developing. While chancres typically develop within 21 days following exposure to the *T. pallidum* bacterium, the small pustule, or pimple, that forms during those initial days is capable of transmitting the syphilis-causing bacterium to a sex partner. The chancre is painless during the weeks it progresses from a small pimple to a complete chancre. By the time 21 days or so have passed, the chancre may develop into a single lesion that is about 2–3 centimeters in diameter, usually painless unless touched by hands, liquids (e.g., water, soap, or urine), or clothing, has a firm base with edges that slope upward into a peak like a pimple. It may appear as a crusted scab and often leaks or slowly oozes a clear or yellowish straw colored liquid called exudate. While most chancres heal on their own within three to six weeks, the surfaces of the chancre, and the liquid that oozes from it, within it, or around it, contain the *T. pallidum* bacterium that can be transmitted to another person and cause syphilis until the lesion is completely healed.

Syphilis, then, is transmitted through sexual activity when a sex partner comes in direct contact with a syphilitic sore, or the "chancre," of an infected person. Transmission of syphilis, further, can occur during unprotected vaginal or anal sex. Oral sex can transmit syphilis also. Once a person has come in contact with the *T. pallidum* bacterium, the first symptoms, if any, typically develop with 21 days but can appear as early as 10 days following exposure or as late as 90 days.

What makes syphilis so concerning is that more and more people are contracting the disease. Additionally, syphilis impacts men and women equally and is affecting people of all races and sexual orientations. For example, in 2014, the CDC reported 63,450 new cases in syphilis, an almost 20,000 increase from previous reports. Even more alarming, the rates of congenital syphilis, or syphilis that is transmitted to a baby by its mother during pregnancy, are steadily rising annually.

Signs and Symptoms

The signs and symptoms of syphilis are elusive and often mistaken for other diseases or conditions. In fact, syphilis has been called the "great pretender" because there are no obvious signs or symptoms that would make someone seek treatment. Additionally, the signs and symptoms of syphilis are so similar to other diseases that it is often the last disease health-care providers consider, and only after all other serious conditions have been explored. However, syphilis typically follows a progression of stages that can last for weeks, months, or even years. Because the symptoms of syphilis can be so long-standing, it is easier to describe syphilis broken down into its specific stages with the specific symptoms that are associated with each stage.

Stages of Syphilis

It is important to distinguish the different stages of syphilis and the symptoms that accompany each stage. These stages include: primary, secondary, and latent (or late stage) syphilis.

1. Primary Stage

The appearance of a single chancre typically marks the primary, or first, stage of syphilis. During this time, the chancre is typically firm, round, and painless. It appears at the location where syphilis entered the body. What complicates identifying syphilis right away is that the chancre is often painless so it goes unnoticed, or it is in a location that makes it difficult to find such as within the vagina or rectum. The chancre lasts about three to six weeks and will heal regardless of whether the person is treated or not. However, proper detection and treatment at this stage is typically successful at curing the disease and removing any of the long-term consequences of the disease. Many people fail to realize they were infected with syphilis and never seek treatment. Outside of the chancre, there are no symptoms such as pain, fever, or discharge that are common with other STDs. Typically, then, the infected person misses the opportunity for adequate treatment and the disease progresses into the secondary stage.

2. Secondary Stage

Once the chancre has healed, syphilis has now been active within the infected person for greater than three to six weeks. New symptoms begin to appear during this stage. Skin rashes, or lesions in the mucous membranes such as sores in the mouth, vagina, or rectum, mark the beginning of the secondary stage of symptoms. In this secondary stage, a rash typically develops on one or more areas of the body. These rashes, then, can occur as the chancre is healing or appear several weeks after the chancre has healed. The characteristic rash of secondary syphilis can appear as non-itching, rough, red or reddish-brown spots on both the palms of the hands or the soles of the feet. However, rashes with a different appearance may occur on other parts of the body and often resemble rashes that are associated with other diseases. Often the rashes associated with secondary syphilis go unnoticed. Conversely, the rash can appear as large, raised, grayish-white lesions, known as condyloma lata, in areas of the body that are typically warm and moist such as the mouth, underarms, or groin areas. In addition to the rashes, other physical symptoms can be present in the secondary stage of syphilis. These symptoms can include fever, sore throat, swollen lymph glands, headache, muscle aches, fatigue, weight loss, or patchy hair loss. However, the symptoms of syphilis can mimic, or be mistaken for, several other conditions or illnesses. Further, the symptoms of secondary syphilis will go away with or without treatment, but the disease remains present in the infected person. While curing syphilis and removing some of the long-term consequences of the disease is still possible during the secondary stage, syphilis tends to go untreated because the symptoms are unnoticed, ignored, or attributed to some other cause. Left untreated, secondary syphilis will progress to the latent, or late, stage of the disease.

3. Latent or Late Stage

The latent stage of syphilis begins when the primary and secondary stage symptoms disappear. Without treatment, the infected person will continue to have syphilis in his or her body despite not having any signs or symptoms. The latent stage is subdivided into two additional stages: early latent syphilis and late latent syphilis. Early latent syphilis is latent syphilis that occurred within the past 12 months. Late latent syphilis describes syphilis where the infection occurred more than 12 months ago. Late latent syphilis, then, can last for years.

The late latent stage of syphilis can develop in about 15 percent of people who were never treated, or not properly treated, for syphilis. The late stages of syphilis can appear 10–20 years after first acquiring the infection. In the late latent stage of syphilis, the disease begins to damage internal organs, specifically the brain, nerves, eyes, heart, blood vessels, and liver. Symptoms of the late latent stage of syphilis, similar to those of the primary and secondary stages, mimic other diseases or conditions. Symptoms during the late latent stage, then, include difficulty with muscle coordination, paralysis, gradual blindness, or dementia. Left untreated, syphilis can eventually lead to damage to key organ systems that may be serious enough to cause death.

Diagnosis

Since the symptoms of syphilis are vague, diagnosing it relies on a thorough heath history and physical examination by a health-care practitioner. During the health interview, the health-care practitioner will inquire about a person's sexual activities and risk for possible exposure to the *T. pallidum* bacterium. When possible, a thorough physical examination with an inspection of the genital areas for the presence of a chancre will follow. A physical examination, however, is not enough; since various signs and symptoms of syphilis are suggestive of other diseases, a health-care practitioner relies instead on specific laboratory blood tests that assist in diagnosing syphilis.

- VDRL (Venereal Disease Research Laboratory) test and RPR (Rapid Plasma Reagent) test. These are simple, inexpensive blood tests that screen a person for syphilis. The important thing to remember is that these two tests are screening tests only. If they come back positive, additional, confirmatory blood tests are required. The VDRL and RPR are not specific only for syphilis and can, therefore, produce false-positive results. However, they are considered adequate for detecting the presence of venereal diseases that require more specific testing.
- Treponemal test. These are specific blood tests that detect the presence of the *T. pallidum* bacterium that cause syphilis. If the VDRL and RPR screen has a positive result, the treponemal tests will, therefore,

confirm if indeed syphilis is present and quantify the amount of *T. pallidum* present within an infected person. A health-care practitioner will use this information, then, to devise an individualized treatment and follow-up plan.

Treatment

Treating syphilis requires an individualized treatment plan that consists of specific antibiotics and a plan for follow-up blood tests to determine if the disease is cured. Fortunately, if found early, the disease is easy to cure. When diagnosed early, a single, one-time injection of antibiotic into a muscle (typically the buttock) is all that is needed to cure the disease. The drug of choice for treating primary, secondary, and often early latent syphilis is an antibiotic in the penicillin family called Benzathine Penicillin G. For some cases of latent or late latent syphilis, Benzathine Penicillin G is given in a series of three individual injections, one injection each week for three weeks. Even though the treatment regimen is simple, it cannot reverse any damage that has already occurred. Similarly, for people who are allergic to, or cannot tolerate, penicillin drugs, more complex regimens are available for health-care practitioners to prescribe that will be equally as effective as Benzathine Penicillin G at curing syphilis. These more complex drug regimens, however, are equally as powerless to reverse any damage that has already occurred because of the progression of syphilis within an infected person's body.

Additional Considerations

One of the ways syphilis is easily transmitted is from a pregnant woman to her baby. According to the CDC, the rates of congenital transmission of syphilis, or syphilis transmitted to a baby by its mother during pregnancy, are on the rise in the United States and internationally. Because the rate of congenital transmission of syphilis is on the rise, the urgency to screen women who are pregnant, or considering becoming pregnant, is high.

Any woman who is considering pregnancy should have a full evaluation by a health-care practitioner prior to becoming pregnant. During this preconception evaluation, a comprehensive health history can be obtained along with testing for the presence of any STDs, including syphilis. With early screening, treatment and follow-up for syphilis can occur that will minimize, or remove any long-term complications for the mother and, therefore, remove the possibility of congenital transmission of syphilis to a baby. Often times, however, women are not screened for STDs or syphilis until they know for certain that they are pregnant. Regardless of the timing, the essential message for any woman is to access health care as soon as possible when pregnancy is desired, confirmed, or suspected.

Another important consideration related to syphilis is the connection of syphilis with HIV infection. Syphilis is transmitted by sexual contact where the bacterium that causes syphilis (*T. pallidum*) enters the body of a sex partner through breaks in the skin or mucous membranes. Since *T. pallidum* can easily enter the body, so, too, can the virus that causes HIV infection through the same break in the skin or mucous membranes. Diseases like syphilis cause open, ulcerative areas on the surfaces of the skin and mucous membranes in the genital areas. Those open areas, in turn, are portals that allow other bacteria or viruses, like HIV, to enter a person's body. Further, during sex, the ulcerative lesions or sores tend to bleed, thereby increasing a person's susceptibility to contracting HIV when the HIV virus comes in contact with oral, vaginal, or rectal mucous membranes during sex. According to the CDC, further, there is a two- to five-fold increased risk of acquiring HIV if exposed to the HIV virus while one is infected with syphilis. Therefore, when a health-care practitioner is evaluating someone with actual or potential syphilis, it is not uncommon and strongly recommended, that a person be screened for HIV as well.

Prevention

Syphilis can be prevented by avoiding exposure to potentially infectious lesions or chancres of an infected sex partner. Therefore, the correct and consistent use of condoms cannot be overemphasized. Since complete abstinence from sexual activity is not a realistic option for most people, the use of barriers like condoms remains the most feasible option for sexually active people. When possible, a long-term, monogamous relationship with a healthy partner minimizes the risk of being infected with syphilis or other STDs. Sexually active people, further, need to remain connected with a health-care practitioner who provides them with at least an annual health evaluation and appropriate screenings for syphilis and other STDs.

Prevention, regular screenings, and early intervention are the only current interventions that have demonstrated success in minimizing the transmission of syphilis. Additionally, urinating with a forceful stream of urine, or washing the genital area immediately after sexual contact are additional measures that have shown to be weakly effective at preventing the transmission of syphilis. Essentially, if any unusual discharge, sores, or rash (especially in the groin area) are noted, one should abstain from any sexual contact and seek evaluation by a health-care practitioner.

Thankfully, syphilis, once treated, does not recur. However, one can be exposed to syphilis from other sex partners and therefore become infected again. Persistence with the use of barrier methods like condoms, and safeguarding one's health through regular check-ups or evaluations by a health-care practitioner, minimizes the threat syphilis poses to a person's health both immediately and for the future.

21. What is Hepatitis B?

The liver is an organ within the body that acts as filter to detoxify harmful substances from the blood as it circulates through the body and produce proteins essential to help blood clot. Hepatitis B is an infection of the liver caused by a virus call the Hepatitis B virus (HBV). Hepatitis B is included with sexually transmitted diseases because sexual contact is one of the primary modes of transmission for Hepatitis B. The Hepatitis B virus, then, is transmitted by blood, semen, or other body fluids from a person infected with the HBV to an uninfected person. The disease itself can be an acute or short-term illness. For many, however, the disease becomes a chronic, long-term condition. Chronic Hepatitis B can have devastating consequences including cirrhosis of the liver, liver cancer, or death.

The Hepatitis B virus requires a portal of entry to pass from an infected person to an uninfected person. HBV is a resilient virus that can survive outside the body for at least seven days and still be capable of causing infection. For most people, sexual contact where the mucous membranes of the penis, vagina, or rectum come in contact with blood, semen, or other body fluid is sufficient to transmit the disease. Additionally, punctures in the skin can serve as a portal of entry for the virus from activities such as sharing needles, syringes or other equipment associated with intravenous drug use, human bites that break through the skin, or sharing items where blood may be present such as shaving equipment or toothbrushes of an infected person. Health-care and public safety workers are at high risk for contracting Hepatitis B from needle stick injuries or from cuts due to sharp surgical instruments. Infected mothers can transmit Hepatitis B to their baby during pregnancy. HBV, however, is not spread through common daily activities such as kissing, hugging, breastfeeding, holding or shaking hands, coughing or sneezing, or sharing utensils. Despite the resiliency of HBV, it is not spread through food, water, insect, or mosquito bites.

Certain groups of people are at higher risk for contracting Hepatitis B. Specifically, sexually active people who are not in long-term monogamous relationships, or those with more than one sex partner during the previous six months, are at highest risk. Further, men who have unprotected anal sex with other men, or people who have repeated sexual contact with someone infected with Hepatitis B are at equally high risk. Outside of sexual activity, intravenous drug users, hemodialysis patients, and residents and staff of facilities serving the developmentally disabled share a burden of risk for contracting Hepatitis B and experiencing symptoms of the disease.

Signs and Symptoms

Signs and symptoms of Hepatitis B vary. Symptoms typically begin an average of 90 days after exposure to the HBV but may occur as early as 60 days after exposure. The most common symptoms are fever, fatigue loss of appetite, nausea, and vomiting. Abdominal pain, typically localized to the right upper quadrant with crampy, aching pain across the stomach, is common. Bowel movements turn to a clay color and urine turns dark. A characteristic yellow tinting of the skin or the white part of the eyes called jaundice may also occur. Symptoms, if any, develop slowly and are often mistaken for other illnesses. However, the person infected with Hepatitis B feels progressively worse, with symptoms lasting anywhere from several weeks to possibly six months. Early diagnosis and treatment, then, helps minimize the symptoms and possibly prevent long-term liver damage.

Diagnosis

Diagnosing Hepatitis B requires a complete medical history and symptom review along with a physical examination by a health-care practitioner. Laboratory blood tests are needed to confirm the diagnosis. Blood tests specific to Hepatitis B include the Hepatitis B Antigen and Hepatitis B Antibody tests. The Hepatitis B Antigen test looks for markers in the blood that are made by the Hepatitis B virus itself; a positive Hepatitis B Antigen test means the HBV is alive in the body. In contrast, the Hepatitis B Antibody test looks for antibodies, or specific proteins made by the body to fight infection. The presence of HBV antibodies means a person, at some point in their lives, was exposed to the Hepatitis B virus, or successfully developed immunity to the disease following the series of vaccinations available to prevent the disease. DNA tests, further, determine if genetic material from the HBV is in the body and aid in determining how severe the infection is or how easily the HBV can spread. In addition to the tests specific for Hepatitis B, the health-care practitioner will also order blood tests that look specifically at how the liver is functioning as an organ (e.g., bilirubin levels, blood clotting tests, and specific liver enzyme levels). Analyzing a urine specimen is also common. Treatment, then, is based upon the severity of the symptoms and how the liver is functioning as an organ determined by the blood tests.

Treatment

For acute Hepatitis B, there is no medication available to kill the Hepatitis B virus. Treatment, then is aimed at controlling the symptoms, providing comfort, rest, and nutrition to allow healing of the liver and preserving the liver's function. Typically, people are advised to stay hydrated, keep fevers down, minimize exertion, and avoid situations that could expose one to other microorganisms and secondary infections. Sexual activity is to be avoided during the acute stage of the illness.

If the Hepatitis B infection becomes chronic, there are several treatment options to help prevent liver damage and possibly the development of liver cancer. Since Hepatitis B is caused by a virus, it can remain in the body indefinitely and cause flare-ups of the hepatitis, damaging the liver more, and often permanently, with each episode. Most people with chronic Hepatitis B, however, can continue to live active lives if they maintain a healthy lifestyle. For some with chronic Hepatitis B, a medication regimen of interferon therapy may be useful to halt the progression of the disease, the growth of HBV in the body, and prevent ongoing, irreversible liver damage.

Interferons occur naturally in the body and are part of the body's natural defense system against infection. When the body is invaded by a virus, for example, HBV, the cells in the body release interferons. These interferons help prevent the virus from infecting new cells, while triggering the immune system to keep producing more interferons to continue the fight against the virus. A synthetic version of interferon was able to be created that mimics the natural interferons that are released from the cells within the body. Injectable interferon, then, boosts the body's natural defenses so it can continue to combat the virus. Interferons are given as a series of injections or intravenous infusions several times per week over a period of several weeks or months.

Prevention

A vaccine was created that effectively provides protection against the Hepatitis B virus. Given as a series of three injections spaced out over time (usually six to eight weeks), the vaccine helps the body develop natural antibodies that destroy the HBV if it enters the body. The vaccine has been so successful that it has become a standard requirement for newborn infants, health-care workers, public safety workers, and first responders. The vaccine, available and recommended to the public, can be administered easily in a health-care practitioner's office or clinic setting.

One of the most effective ways to prevent Hepatitis B is through the proper and consistent use of condoms. Since semen, blood, or other body fluids, including those found in the vagina and rectum, come in direct contact with susceptible mucous membranes, the risk of transmitting HBV, or other microorganisms, is high. Condoms, then, contain the semen or seminal fluid within them while protecting the penis and the mucous membranes of the vagina or rectum. Condoms should be changed regularly during repeated episodes of sexual activity and not reused or shared. Outside of sexual activity, there are also public health requirements that prevent people from transmitting the HBV by accident; people with Hepatitis B, or a history of carrying the HBV, are not permitted to be blood, organ, or sperm donors. Further, people with Hepatitis B infection or known to carry the HBV should not share personal items such as razors or toothbrushes.

Since the liver is one of the major organs within the body that regulates important bodily functions. There are no dietary supplements, herbal preparations, or over-the-counter medications that specifically target the liver. Therefore, a healthy diet that is balanced with proteins and nutrients helps maintain the liver's integrity. Similarly, alcohol intake can damage the liver; even small amounts of alcohol consumed regularly will begin to break down the liver's ability to filter blood and detoxify harmful substances. For optimal liver health, then, one should maintain minimal alcohol intake. Coupled with diet and a decreased alcohol intake, exercise balanced with rest allows the liver to maximally perform its filtering functions and helps the liver resist infection and damage that occur because of inflammation. A person diagnosed with Hepatitis B, or found to have the HBV, will have ongoing monitoring and follow-up by a health-care practitioner, including regular blood tests to evaluate the liver's function.

22. What is Hepatitis C?

Hepatitis C is a contagious liver disease that ranges in severity from a mild illness lasting a few weeks to a serious, lifelong illness that destroys the liver. The liver is an organ that acts as a filter to detoxify harmful substances in the body, process blood as it circulates through the body, and produce proteins essential to help blood clot. Hepatitis C is similar to Hepatitis B in several ways: both are caused by a virus, both cause similar symptoms, both are spread through contact with infected blood, semen, and body fluids, and both can be an acute or chronic illness. Hepatitis C and B, however, differ. The causative organism for Hepatitis C is a particularly resilient virus known as the Hepatitis C virus (HCV) and, unlike Hepatitis B, there is no vaccine currently available to prevent the disease.

Hepatitis C, like Hepatitis B, is spread primarily when infected blood comes in contact with mucous membranes of an uninfected person, or when the protective barrier of the skin is broken or punctured thereby allowing the Hepatitis C virus to enter the body. While most people in the United States become infected with Hepatitis C by sharing needles or other equipment used for intravenous drug use, sexual activity can serve as a mechanism to transmit Hepatitis C from an infected person to an uninfected person. With Hepatitis C, further, incidence of the disease has been linked to tattooing when people opt to not use licensed, commercial tattooing establishments and home, or nonprofessional, methods to create a tattoo. People who engage in rough vaginal or anal sex, have multiple sex partners, already have an STD or are HIV-positive are at particular risk for contracting Hepatitis C. Similar to Hepatitis B, blood, semen, or other bodily fluids can come in contact with the mucous membranes of the penis, vagina, or rectum and transmit the Hepatitis C virus. The groups at highest risk for Hepatitis C, however, are similar to those at risk for Hepatitis B: sexually active people who are not in long-term monogamous relationships, or those with more than one sex partner during the previous six months, men who have unprotected anal sex with other men, people who have unprotected sex with a partner already infected with Hepatitis C virus, intravenous drug users, hemodialysis patients, and those sharing razors or toothbrushes with people who are infected with the Hepatitis C virus. Further, mothers can transmit Hepatitis C to their unborn baby during pregnancy. Like Hepatitis B, Hepatitis C is not transmitted by casual contact such as kissing, hugging, shaking or holding hands, breastfeeding, or sharing utensils. Hepatitis C is not known to be spread through food, water, insects, or mosquito bites. Signs and symptoms of Hepatitis C, further, are as elusive as those linked to Hepatitis B.

Signs and Symptoms

Approximately, 70 to 80 percent of people with acute Hepatitis C have no symptoms of the disease. If symptoms occur, they typically appear six to seven weeks after exposure; some symptoms appear as early as two weeks to as late as six months after exposure. When symptoms are present, they can resemble the symptoms of Hepatitis B and include fever, fatigue, loss of appetite, nausea, and vomiting. Like Hepatitis B, abdominal pain is common but the pain and discomfort is diffuse across the abdomen with tenderness in the right upper and middle quadrants of the abdomen. Like Hepatitis B, bowel movements are clay colored and the urine turns dark. Jaundice, or yellowing of the skin and the white portion of the eye, are common. However, since the majority of symptoms of Hepatitis C are subtle, many people with the disease are unaware they have it and continue to pass the disease from partner to partner. Early diagnosis, then, is essential to minimize long-term damage from the disease.

Diagnosis

A thorough medical history review and a physical examination by a health-care practitioner is required to make a definitive diagnosis of Hepatitis C. Additionally, the health-care practitioner will use laboratory blood tests to assist in making the diagnosis. The Hepatitis C Antibody test, or the Anti-HCV test, looks for antibodies against the Hepatitis C virus. A negative, or nonreactive, Hepatitis C antibody test means that a person does not have Hepatitis C. However, if the Hepatitis C antibody test is positive, or reactive, additional blood tests are needed to confirm a diagnosis of Hepatitis C. Since exposure to Hepatitis C at any time in one's life will cause the body to create antibodies, an additional test is needed to discover if someone is currently infected with Hepatitis C. The RNA (ribonucleic acid) test, or PCR (polymerase chain reaction) test, is done to identify if genetic material from the Hepatitis C virus is in the body. If the RNA or PCR test is negative, the person does not have Hepatitis C. However, if the RNA or PCR test is positive, a person has active Hepatitis C disease and needs additional blood tests to determine if the liver is functioning properly. Treatment, then, is based upon the symptoms a person has and how well the liver is functioning.

Treatment

There is no cure for Hepatitis C. Acute Hepatitis C, if found early, responds well to conventional treatments aimed at healing the infection, protecting the liver from damage, and providing relief of any symptoms. Like Hepatitis B, the Hepatitis C virus cannot be destroyed by antibiotics and can remain within the body indefinitely. Treatment for acute Hepatitis C, then, involves controlling the symptoms a person is experiencing and providing rest, comfort, and nutrition to allow healing of the liver to occur. Typically, people are advised to stay hydrated, keep fevers down, minimize exertion, and avoid situations that could expose one to other microorganisms and secondary infections. Sexual activity is to be avoided during the acute stage of the illness.

If Hepatitis C becomes chronic, new drug regimens have been discovered that have shown to be effective for treating chronic Hepatitis C. Known as Hepatitis C virus inhibitor therapies, these drugs essentially enter the Hepatitis C virus itself and prevent it from replicating, thereby decreasing the number and strength of the Hepatitis C virus in the body. While advances in drug therapy for both acute and chronic Hepatitis C continue to be made, there remains no definitive cure for the disease. No vaccine, further, is available to prevent it. Prevention, then, focuses on minimizing exposure to the Hepatitis C virus and keeping the liver, and the immune system overall, resilient to fight off infections.

Prevention

Since no vaccine is currently available to prevent Hepatitis C, steps should be taken to avoid exposure to the Hepatitis C virus. Sexual activity remains a primary mode of transmission for Hepatitis C. The proper and consistent use of condoms, then, is an effective way of preventing the spread of the Hepatitis C virus. Since semen, blood, or other body fluids, including those found in the vagina and rectum, come in direct contact with susceptible mucous membranes, the risk of transmitting HCV, or other microorganisms, is high. Condoms, then, contain the semen or seminal fluid within them while protecting the penis and the mucous membranes of the vagina or rectum. Condoms should be changed regularly during repeated episodes of sexual activity and not reused or shared. Outside of sexual activity, there are also public health requirements that prevent people from transmitting the HCV by accident; people with Hepatitis C, or a history of carrying the HCV, are not permitted to be blood, organ, or sperm donors. Further, people with Hepatitis C infection or known to carry the HCV should not share personal items such as razors or toothbrushes.

Like Hepatitis B, protecting the liver from damage by an acute or chronic Hepatitis C infection and maintaining its optimal function as a filtering organ is essential. There are no dietary supplements, herbal preparations, or over-the-counter medications that specifically target the liver. Therefore, a healthy diet that is balanced with proteins and nutrients helps maintain the liver's integrity. Similarly, alcohol intake can damage the liver; even small amounts of alcohol consumed regularly will begin to break down the liver's ability to filter blood and detoxify harmful substances. For optimal liver health, then, one should maintain minimal alcohol intake. Coupled with diet and a decreased alcohol intake, exercise balanced with rest allows the liver to maximally perform its filtering functions and helps the liver resist infection and damage that occur because of inflammation. A person diagnosed with Hepatitis C, or found to have the HCV, will have ongoing monitoring and follow-up by a health-care practitioner, including regular blood tests to evaluate the liver's function.

23. What is HIV?

One of the most infamous and potentially devastating of all STDs is human immunodeficiency virus, or HIV. Over the past two decades, the incidence of HIV has steadily increased and now affects men and women equally, regardless of age, race, sexual orientation, or socioeconomic status. Indeed, HIV has become a worldwide epidemic and, therefore, a global concern. Fortunately, advances in scientific research have led to the creation of various drug regimens that not only halt the progression of the disease but also work to prevent the disease in individuals who are at increased risk of contracting HIV. Despite the advances, knowledge about HIV and safe-sex practices remain the most powerful tools to prevent contracting this potentially deadly virus.

HIV is a virus that attacks a person's immune system, or the body's natural defense system. Both the virus, and the disease it causes, then, is called HIV. What complicates HIV, similar to other viruses, for example, herpes, is that there is no treatment to kill off the virus or a cure for the illness or infections caused by it; once a person contracts HIV, they will have it for life.

HIV belongs to a viral genus, lentivirus, and is part of a viral family known as *retroviridae*, or retroviruses. Lentiviruses have a unique characteristic: they infect a host and are responsible for long-duration illnesses with a long incubation period. With HIV, it is not uncommon for a person to carry HIV for years without any symptoms, but the person will carry the virus for life. Because these types of viruses are often so virulent and highly infective, they are the cause of the majority of HIV infections globally.

Once HIV enters the body, it goes directly to the cells within the immune system that work to fight off infections or illnesses, known as the CD4 cells and the T cells. Unlike other viruses or microorganisms, HIV attaches to, or becomes part of, the host's T cells. HIV can spread from cell to cell easily. For example, an infected T cell can come in contact with the cellular fluid of a noninfected T cell and transmit the virus to the unaffected cell through a process called cell-to-cell spread. More commonly, cells transmit HIV to each other by direct contact within the body. There are areas in the body, for example, the lymph tissue, where CD4 cells are numerous and densely packed; cells touching cells, then, is unavoidable, and HIV can be easily spread. What is important to keep in mind is that one cell does not transfer HIV to another in this process; each infected cell contributes a portion of HIV to the uninfected cell while retaining a significant portion of HIV to itself. Following cell-to-cell contact, then, two cells are now infected with HIV. HIV, then, will continue to grow and replicate within the infected cells and will continue to spread the virus to other cells through contact.

Transmission

HIV requires a bodily fluid to pass from one person to another. Therefore, HIV lives in:

- Blood
- Semen of pre-seminal fluid (i.e., "pre-cum")
- Vaginal fluids
- Rectal fluids or anal mucous
- Breast milk

The one body fluid where HIV is not found is saliva. However, given the number of body fluids where HIV can live, it is easy to transmit the virus from an infected person to another. The primary modes of transmission, then, include unprotected sexual activity (i.e., sex without using a condom), passing HIV to a baby by its mother during pregnancy, sharing needles during intravenous drug use, contaminated blood transfusions, or receiving an organ transplant from an infected person.

To become infected, bodily fluids from an infected person need to gain access to the bloodstream of an uninfected person. This happens, typically, through a mucous membrane such as the lining of the vagina, rectum, the opening of the penis, or in the mouth. Additionally, breaks in the skin like cuts, bites, or scrapes can serve as entry points for HIV into the bloodstream of an uninfected person. Sexual activity, however, remains a primary mechanism for the transmission of HIV.

Oral sex poses unique opportunities for transmission of HIV also. Since HIV can live in pre-seminal fluid, HIV can be transmitted to an uninfected person if the pre-seminal fluid of an infected person comes in contact with sores, lesions, or open areas on the lips, gums, or oral surfaces of an uninfected person, transmission can occur. Ejaculating into the mouth, further, puts an uninfected person at risk. Swallowing semen immediately, or ejaculating deep into the back of the throat, does not minimize the risk of transmitting HIV.

Vaginal intercourse between and man and a woman can put both partners at risk for transmitting HIV. Rubbing the penis across the opening of the vagina or rectum exposes both partners to each other's fluids or secretions. Sex, or intercourse, is typically a vigorous activity with frequent thrusting movements in and out of the vagina; these movements can cause irritation, abrasions, or small tears to the inner lining of the vagina that can then become a portal of entry for HIV. Similarly, for men, unprotected vaginal intercourse allows any of the vaginal fluids or secretions to easily enter a man's body through the opening of the penis. Ejaculating into the vagina, then, exposes all of the vaginal surfaces, including the cervix of the uterus, to a large amount of fluid at one time that may contain HIV. Douching or swabbing out the vagina after sex is useless and will not prevent the transmission of HIV. For men, urinating after sex with a forceful stream will not minimize or prevent the transmission of HIV.

Anal sex, regardless if it is sex between hetero- or homosexual couples, carries similar risks of transmitting HIV. Since the rectum and anus contain more constrictive-type muscles than the vagina, the anus, and the rectal opening are tighter and therefore more highly susceptible to tearing or breaking down during vigorous sexual activity. Further, the rectum itself is often an area with frequently irritated skin caused by wiping after a bowel movement or from the irritation of hemorrhoids or tight clothing. Any of these surfaces, then, are susceptible to exposure to HIV, more so if pre-seminal fluid is present or if ejaculation of semen occurs across the anus or within the rectum occurs.

Breaks in skin, further, make people vulnerable to exposure to HIV. Bites to the body, whether through playful exchange during sex or through physical aggression, lead to breaks in the skin that make one susceptible to HIV if they are exposed to infected blood or body fluids. Transmission, then, is not isolated solely to sexual activity or intercourse.

Pregnancy is another example where HIV is transmitted outside of direct sexual activity. An HIV positive woman, therefore, can transmit HIV to her unborn baby regardless of the father's HIV status. Throughout pregnancy, the uterus is an environment that not only nurtures and grows a baby until the time of delivery, but also protects a baby from injury or harm. The placenta serves as a protective barrier for the baby from most harmful microorganisms or substances that a mother may ingest or be exposed to. With HIV, the protective mechanisms of the placenta are weakened, thereby making the baby susceptible to contact with HIV. Even if the mother is healthy despite being HIV positive, the process of delivering the baby through the birth canal and vagina exposes the mucous membranes of the baby to direct contact with the secretions, fluids, and blood of the mother's vagina and rectum. Lastly, the baby can be exposed to breast milk containing HIV following delivery. Because transmission of HIV during pregnancy is on the rise, rigorous screening of all pregnant women, or women considering pregnancy, is recommended. Additionally, the preferred method of delivery for these babies is via Cesarean section and breastfeeding after delivery is highly discouraged.

Sexual activity and childbirth are not the only ways to contract, or transmit, HIV. Illicit drug use, environmental conditions, or specific medical situations make one susceptible to HIV also. Intravenous (IV) drug use continues to plague society and remains another mode of transmitting HIV. Additionally, certain occupations make exposure to HIV unavoidable, for example, health-care workers, emergency responders, police, or corrections personnel. Lastly, and not as common in modern times in areas with advanced health care, transmission through blood transfusions from HIV positive donors or where organs have been transplanted from HIV positive donors remain a viable, potential source of transmitting HIV to uninfected people.

Risk

HIV can affect anyone, regardless of sexual orientation, race, ethnicity, gender, or age. However, certain groups are at a high risk for HIV based on specific lifestyle activities or societal circumstances. These include women, gay and bisexual men, people of color, older and younger people, and those incarcerated.

Women represent one of the highest groups, internationally, affected by HIV. According to the CDC, almost one out of every four women in the United States is HIV positive. Most contracted HIV through heterosexual activity. The primary cause of these increased numbers is the amount of unprotected sex women engage in. However, most women engage in unprotected sex with partners who are uncertain of their HIV status. Similarly, HIV infection among transgender women is on the rise. According to recent studies by the CDC, an astonishing 28 percent of transgender women reported being HIV positive, with more black/African American and Latino transgender women reporting the highest rates of HIV.

Gay and bisexual men remain the largest group affected by HIV in the United States. Black/African American men, followed by Latino men, bear the highest reported rates of HIV currently. Sexual behaviors and activity remain the biggest risk factor for gay and bisexual men, with many practicing unprotected anal and oral sex. Additionally, many gay and bisexual men, despite the availability of testing, have no knowledge of their HIV status. Further, a noticeable trend among younger gay and bisexual men is the deliberate choice to have unprotected anal and/or oral sex ("bare backing") despite the increased availability of condoms. Moreover, gay and bisexual men report an increase in the frequency of unprotected sexual encounters and admit to a variety of partners, including women.

People of color and those of diverse ethnic backgrounds are emerging as another large group who are HIV positive. African Americans are the racial/ethnic group most affected by HIV in the United States followed by Latinos. Multiple factors have been explored and implicated for the rise of HIV among both African Americans and Latinos. These include the increased poverty rate among African Americans and Latinos that is linked to limited access to high quality health care, HIV testing, and prevention education. Further, these groups have been found to bear a unique burden of stigmatization, discrimination, and fear surrounding HIV testing and living with an HIV diagnosis.

HIV is now becoming more prevalent among two groups: younger and older people. According to the CDC, young people aged 13 to 24 accounted for more than 1 in 5 new HIV diagnoses. Young, African American, and Hispanic/Latino men are especially affected. On the opposite end of the life span, older adults with HIV are increasing in numbers also. The reason for this is two-fold: (1) improvements in treatment for HIV have allowed HIV positive people to live longer, healthier lives, and (2) older people are continuing to participate in activities, like their younger counterparts, that continue to expose them to transmitting or contracting HIV. According to the CDC, in 2012, the largest number of newly diagnosed cases of HIV among adults over aged 50, with people over age 55 accounting for one-fourth of all Americans living with HIV. Specific chronic conditions such as heart or kidney disease, along with various cancers, can complicate treatment plans for particular older adults or make certain plans ineffective. Further, because certain medical conditions mask or mimic other diseases, HIV may go unnoticed or unsuspected, thereby delaying diagnosis in older adults until the later stages of the disease.

Another group that is often overlooked is current or previously incarcerated men and women. HIV has become a serious health issue among correctional facilities. While many of those incarcerated contracted HIV prior to being in prison, the correctional facility is often where the incarcerated person is tested for, and diagnosed with, HIV for the first time. Of the current incarcerated population, the majority of inmates are black, African American, and Latino men and women compared to the overall incarcerated population. Certain high-risk behaviors have been identified among current and previously incarcerated people. For example, unprotected sex with various partner or intravenous drug use prior to incarceration, and continuing those behaviors while incarcerated.

Signs and Symptoms

There are no obvious symptoms of HIV. In fact, many signs and symptoms of HIV are shared with other diseases and those are often ruled out first before making a definitive diagnosis of HIV. The symptoms of HIV, then, vary depending on the individual and what stage (i.e., early, latent, or AIDS) the disease is in.

Early Stage

In the early stages of HIV, a person may experience a flu-like illness within two to four weeks after HIV infection. Most people, however, will have no symptoms in this stage and are often unaware they have HIV at all. For those who have symptoms, they often experience such things as fever, chills, night sweats, muscle aches, and a pale pink to pale red rash on various parts of the body. One may also experience a sore throat, swollen glands, increased fatigue, and mouth sores during this stage. These symptoms can last anywhere from a few days to several weeks. Since these symptoms mimic other common conditions, most people will endure them until they pass and mistakenly assume they had a "bad cold" or "the flu."

Latent Stage

Once the symptoms have resolved, HIV will go into clinical latency stage. During this time, HIV is still active in one's body but it reproduces at very low levels. People may experience no further symptoms but are still capable of transmitting HIV to uninfected partners. If a person is diagnosed properly, however, antiretroviral therapy, or ART, can keep the disease in check and potentially provide decades of health for a person with HIV. While a person can still transmit HIV to an uninfected person, antiretroviral therapy can minimize the disease progression and suppress any viral activity (i.e., low levels of the virus will be detected in the blood).

AIDS

HIV left unopposed by antiretroviral medications will, over time, weaken the body's immune system. The weakened immune system, then, leads to the late stages of HIV infection known as acquired immune deficiency syndrome, or AIDS. Symptoms of AIDS vary but may include rapid weight loss, recurring fevers with profuse night sweats, extreme fatigue, prolonged swollen glands, persistent diarrhea, sores in the mouth, genitals, or rectum that do not heal, or purple to reddish-brown blotchy rashes on or under the skin. Since AIDS destroys the immune system, a person with AIDS is susceptible to other types of infections. These opportunistic infections can be severe and possibly cause death. The symptoms of AIDS, then, are also the symptoms of other acute diseases; the only definitive way to determine if the symptoms are truly indicative of AIDS is through specific testing.

Diagnosis

The most common test available for detecting HIV is a test, called an immunoassay, which looks for antibodies that one's body produces against HIV. This immunoassay test can be done as a traditional blood test in a laboratory or as a rapid test performed on oral fluid (not saliva) at a testing site or clinic. While rapid tests are convenient, provide answers quickly, and can be done on multiple people at one event, the level of antibody found in oral fluids is lower than it is in blood. Blood-based laboratory tests, then, detect HIV sooner after exposure than the rapid HIV tests.

What is important to point out is that the immunoassay tests, regardless if done as a blood-based lab test or as a rapid test on oral fluid, are only screening tests. They are not definitive or confirmatory for HIV; rather, they indicate if additional testing is needed to confirm a diagnosis of HIV. All immunoassay tests that are positive require a follow-up test to confirm if the person is, indeed, HIV positive.

Follow-up testing is done through a blood-based laboratory test that looks specifically at, and differentiates, antibodies created in response to exposure to human immunodeficiency virus. This test, then, confirms if the antibodies are HIV-1 or from HIV-2 (a rare form of the virus not commonly found in North America). There is also the Western blot or indirect immunofluorescence assay that uses a blood-based lab test to detect antibodies to HIV. Additionally, another blood-based lab test called the HIV-1 nucleic acid test looks for the presence of virus directly.

Currently, there are two home tests one can purchase and perform on themselves at home. One is the Home Access HIV-1 Test System that involves pricking one's finger to collect a blood sample. That blood sample is sent to a licensed laboratory and results are often available the next day. If the test is positive, the laboratory performs a follow-up test on the same specimen of blood. The person providing the specimen remains anonymous throughout the whole process. The person obtains his or her results by calling into the laboratory; the manufacturer, in turn, provides confidential counseling and referral for treatment for anyone who purchases and uses a home-testing kit. While accurate, the tests conducted on a blood specimen collected in the home find infections later compared to blood-based laboratory tests but detect infections sooner compared to tests done in the home with oral fluids.

The second home test is the OraQuick In-Home HIV test. This test involves one swabbing his or her mouth to collect oral fluids and using a kit to test it. Results are available in 20 minutes. If the test is positive, the person needs additional testing to confirm HIV. Like the Home Access HIV-1 Test, the manufacturer of the OraQuick In-Home HIV test provides confidential counseling and referral to follow-up testing sites. The level of antibody is lower in oral fluids than in blood; oral fluid tests, then, find infection later compared to traditional blood-based laboratory tests. While the in-home oral fluid test is convenient and provides an answer quickly, up to 1 in 12 people may receive a false negative result with the in-home test. Other home HIV tests exist and new ones continue to emerge on the market; it is important to verify that whichever test one uses is Food and Drug Administration (FDA) approved.

Frequency of Testing

How often a person is tested for HIV depends on multiple factors, including the person's lifestyle, risk factors, and overall health status. Currently, the CDC recommends health practitioners testing everyone between the ages of 13 and 64 at least once as a part of routine health care. In other words, one should have an HIV test during annual, routine medical check-ups along with any other routine blood or urine tests that are used to determine health status.

Outside of annual testing, some specific lifestyle change or at risk behaviors may trigger a health-care practitioner to recommend testing for HIV on a more frequent basis. Testing is individualized to the person so one should be honest and up-front with his or her health-care practitioner when answering questions about sexual activity, risky behaviors, or life-style choices. Questions a health-care provider may ask include:

- Have you had sex with someone who is HIV positive or whose HIV status you did not know since your last HIV test?
- Have you injected drugs (or steroids, silicone, or hormones) and shared injecting equipment (such as syringes or needles) with others?
- Have you been diagnosed and treated for any STDs?
- Have you had unprotected sex?
- Are you engaging in homosexual or bisexual intercourse?
- Are you having sex with anyone who would answer "Yes" to any of these questions or with someone whose health and sexual history you do not know?

If a woman or a couple is planning to become pregnant, an HIV test should be performed prior to becoming pregnant or during the first trimester if already pregnant. The CDC recommends another HIV test during the third trimester for women at high risk for HIV or for women who live in areas where there are high rates of HIV infection among pregnant women or among women aged 15 to 44. In some states, further, if a mother refuses to be tested, or does not receive HIV testing during pregnancy, her infant will be tested for HIV at birth.

Disclosing HIV Test Results

In the United States, a person's medical information is protected by specific privacy rules under the Health Insurance Portability and Accountability Act (HIPAA) of 1996. HIV test results fall under the same privacy rules. However, not all HIV-testing sites are bound by HIPAA regulations; one should inquire about privacy rules of a potential site as well as those surrounding the test results. Most states, therefore, offer testing that is both confidential and anonymous. Some, however, only offer confidential testing services.

Confidential testing means that your name and any other identifying information (for example, your address or date of birth) will be attached to your test results. Your results, then, become part of a medical record. People who are part of a health-care team involved in your care, and possibly your insurance company, then, can have access to your results. However, the health-care team and your insurance company alike cannot share your information, or divulge test results, without your written permission. With confidential testing, in most states if the HIV test, or test for an STD, is positive, the test results and your name are reported to the state and local health department to allow estimates of HIV or STD incidence rates. The state, in turn, removes all identifying information and shares the information with the CDC so national statistics can be collected. Anonymous testing, in contrast, means there are no identifiable ties between you and your test results. People taking an anonymous HIV test get a unique identifier (typically a series of numbers or a combination of numbers and letters) that allows them access to their test results.

Many states, however, have partner notification laws that obligate you, or your health-care practitioner, to tell any sex partners or needle-sharing partners about your status if your HIV test is positive. In some states, further, if you are HIV positive and do not disclose this information to your partners, you could be charged with a crime. Some health departments require health-care practitioners to report the name of your sex and needle-sharing partners if that information is known. Additionally, some states have laws that require clinic staff to notify a third party (e.g., the health department or other agency) if they know that someone in the community is at significant risk to be exposed to HIV from a clinic patient that is known to be HIV positive. Under the *duty to warn*, any health department that receives funding through the Ryan White HIV/AIDS program is required to show "good faith" efforts to notify the marriage partners of patients with HIV/AIDS. To find out the laws of specific states, refer to www.AIDS.gov.

Treatment

Since HIV is a virus, there is no cure. Therefore, a person will have the virus in his or her body for a lifetime. However, advances in research and science have led to the development of a group of medications that slow, or halt, the progression of HIV. Since HIV is a lentivirus that belongs to the group called retroviridiae, the specific medications for HIV are known as antiretroviral therapy, or ART. The goal of ART, then, is to control the virus so a person can live a longer, healthier life and lower that person's risk of transmitting HIV to others. There is not one specific ART drug. Instead, a combination of drugs, called a regimen, is used. Some of these drugs, currently, have been combined into single pills. The single pills, however, can be costly. Regardless, a regimen that is individualized to each person is expected to be taken every day as prescribed.

The drugs for HIV, then, prevent HIV from multiplying (i.e., HIV copying itself into uninfected cells) in order to reduce the amount of HIV in the body. With less HIV in the body, the immune system has a better chance of fighting off infections because it is not being destroyed by the virus. HIV is still in the body; however, a number of cells, with the help of ART, remain uninfected with HIV and can continue to fight infections or even cancers. Additionally, if the amount of HIV is reduced in the body, there is then less chance to transmit HIV to an uninfected person. ART, then, is recommended for all people with HIV, regardless of how long they have had the virus or how healthy they are. Without ART, HIV will continue to spread throughout the body, attack the immune system, and eventually progress to AIDS.

While ART is recommended for everyone infected with HIV because it helps people live longer, healthier lives, starting ART depends upon several factors. Specifically, starting ART is dependent upon a person's CD4 count (i.e., the amount of specific CD4 lymphocytes in a sample of blood that indicates how well the immune system is working and how HIV, overall, is progressing). Additionally, starting ART is dependent upon whether the person had any other diseases or conditions, HIV-related illnesses, AIDS, or pregnancy. Above all, starting ART depends upon whether the person is committed to a lifelong course of therapy, monitoring, and follow-up by a health-care practitioner.

ART, as a lifelong commitment, requires people to take their prescribed regimen exactly as it is ordered. Certain combinations of ART require additional lifestyle modifications such as eliminating alcohol, following a special diet, or taking the medications at specific times of the day. Some ART may interact poorly with medications used for other conditions, so other drug regimens for chronic, and sometimes acute, conditions may need to be modified. It is important, then, for people taking ART to alert any health-care practitioner, including dentists or other specialists who might prescribe them medication, what specific drug or regimen one is taking. This information helps prevent complications with, or interruptions in, the prescribed regimen.

Prevention

The only absolute way to avoid contracting HIV is to avoid any and all circumstances where transmission of the virus can occur. This strategy, while logical, is not always feasible in today's society. To that end, there are some safeguards people can employ to minimize their chances of becoming infected with HIV. These include testing, safer-sex practices, maintaining overall good health, or the use of pre-exposure prophylactic medications.

First, get tested. Knowing your HIV status lets you protect yourself from being exposed to situations that could further weaken your immune system if you are HIV positive. Further, knowing your status lets you begin treatment, such as ART, sooner to slow or halt the progression of HIV within your body. Knowing your HIV status also lets you protect someone else from being infected through the use of safer-sex methods like condoms. Depending on the number of sex partners you have, or how risky your other behaviors are in your lifestyle, may warrant more frequent testing. An HIV test, then, is a sort of snapshot of the current moment in time; a negative HIV test does not mean it will always be negative with future tests. Be honest with yourself, and future partners, about your habits, lifestyle, or practices and incorporate HIV testing as indicated.

Second, condoms remain the superior form of protection against HIV. Other forms of contraception prevent unwanted pregnancy but do nothing to prevent HIV. Birth control pills, intrauterine devices (IUDs), diaphragms, spermicidal gels, and permanent sterilization have no impact on HIV. Contact with body fluids of an infected person needs to be avoided, so both male and female condoms are the only available products that contain body fluids within them. Further, both male and female condoms cover the skin and mucous membrane surfaces that body fluids could come in contact with, acting as a protective barrier during its use. While condoms can break or leak, especially if they are used improperly or are the wrong size, the majority of condoms available today are made of a high quality, durable material that is designed to withstand vigorous vaginal, anal, and oral sexual activity. Proper usage, then, is key.

Condoms are single-use only. They should be changed regularly depending on the length of the sexual activity session. Condoms should never be washed and reused; they should be thrown out after each use. The male condom should fit snugly along the penis with no air pockets noticeable and unrolled fully to the base of the penis. Most male condoms have a space at the tip to collect ejaculated semen; that pocket or space needs to be visible and not stretched out while putting on a condom. Male condoms come in a variety of styles, but it is important to use one that completely covers the penis snugly and that does not roll up or down loosely, or create pockets or air bubbles, while in use. Female condoms, in contrast, are inserted into the vagina and unrolled outward to the vaginal opening. The edges of the condom extend, or hang over, the vaginal opening, essentially forming a bag inside the vagina. When fitted properly, all surfaces of the vagina are covered. While the female condom is simple to use, many women, and men, dislike the feel of the female condom and find it dampens their sexual experience. Many women further, dislike having to interrupt foreplay to insert the female condom, or find it too messy or cumbersome to manage. The female condom, however, cannot be used for anal sex. Regardless of which style or type is chosen, condoms protect the mucous membrane surfaces from exposure to, or as a point of entry for, HIV.

Third, good health contributes greatly to preventing HIV or minimizes its progression. When one follows a proper diet, maintains an ideal body weight, and exercises regularly, the body remains nourished and resilient. Further, maintaining overall health sustains the immune system to ward off illness and prevents lesions, sores, or ulcers from developing within the mouth, vagina, or rectum. Tissues of the body, such as those within the mouth, vagina, or rectum, are less likely to tear or break when maintained in a healthy condition that comes only from proper nutrition with balanced rest and exercise. Stress, additionally, can weaken a person's immune system but a body that is healthy is better able to minimize the impact of stress.

What has been gaining popularity to prevent HIV is PrEP, or Pre Exposure Prophylaxis. PrEP is designed for people who are at substantial risk of getting HIV to have a reliable means to prevent it through the use of medication. PrEP is a pill available only by a prescription that is a combination of two drugs: tenofovir and emtricitabine, called "Truvada" on the current market. When someone is at risk for being exposed to HIV through sex or injecting drugs, PrEP works to keep HIV from establishing a permanent infection. Like any of the drug regimens for HIV, PrEP requires someone to take it consistently and as prescribed. When taken consistently, however, PrEP has been shown to greatly reduce the incidence of HIV in certain high-risk groups.

PrEP, like the other drugs for HIV, requires monitoring and follow-up by a health-care practitioner. An HIV test is needed prior to starting PrEP to ensure one does not have HIV already, and then follow-up HIV tests at regular intervals (e.g., every three to six months) is also required. PrEP can also be costly and may not be covered by some insurance plans; assistance may be available depending on a person's circumstances or where they live.

PrEP is not meant to replace any of the other prevention strategies for HIV. Further, PrEP does not give one protection from any of the other STDs; therefore, condoms should continue to be used for all sexual activity. PrEP, combined with the proper and consistent use of condoms greatly reduces one's chances of HIV infection compared to either method used alone.

24. What is bacterial vaginosis?

Bacterial vaginosis, or BV, is not an STD in the traditional sense. It is not contagious, nor does it cause long-term side effects or damage. However, having sex increases a woman's chance of getting BV and the condition affects only women. The vagina is full of bacteria and microorganism that are harmless to a woman. These normally occurring microorganisms, or "good" flora, regulate the environment within the vagina. They prevent other harmful bacteria from growing, or some infections, especially yeast, from occurring. The balance of bacteria, however, can change easily. Common things that disrupt the natural bacteria in the vagina are antibiotic use, stress, having a menstrual period, hygiene products like douches, hormonal changes, diet changes, tampon use, or sex.

Sexual activity can alter the pH level inside the vagina. pH is a measure of how acidic, or how alkaline or basic, an environment is. In the vagina, the normal pH ranges tend to lean more toward an acidic environment (pH = 3.5 to 4.5, where typical pH is considered neutral at 7.0). During sex, lubricants, spermicides, a condom, or the skin of the penis itself can neutralize the normally acidic environment of the vagina. Further, if a couple is practicing unprotected sex, ejaculated semen, which has an alkaline pH of 7.1 to 8, can neutralize the acidic environment of the vagina and allow other organisms, like the bacteria that cause BV, to grow. Since BV relies on an alkaline vaginal environment, only women can contract BV. Male sex partners do not manifest the disease nor do they spread BV from partner to partner. BV, however, may be spread between female sex partners.

BV is caused by anaerobic bacteria, *Gardnerella vaginalis*, or G. *vaginalis*. As the lactobacilli common in the vagina die off because they cannot survive if the vaginal environment is too alkaline, there is no longer protection to prevent anaerobic bacteria, like G. *vaginalis* from multiplying. While many women's bodies will auto-regulate themselves over time and restore their own natural balance of useful, harmless microorganisms in the vagina, when BV grows and multiplies it becomes too numerous inside the vagina and prevents the "good" microorganisms from ever repopulating. Women with BV will not be aware of the changes occurring in the vagina. However, BV has unique signs and symptoms that cause women to seek a medical evaluation by a health-care practitioner.

Signs and Symptoms

The most notorious sign of BV is the presence of a foul-smelling, fishy, odor from the vagina. The odor is worse immediately after sexual activity but lingers for hours or days after. Soaps, perfumes, or powders are not effective at covering up or eliminating the odor. In fact, frequent showering, tub baths, douches, or cleaning the vagina with soap makes the condition worse. Some women will notice a white to gray discharge on their underpants, pads, or panty liners. Sometimes the discharge is irritating and causes itching at the vaginal opening. When a woman with BV has her menstrual period, the odor, irritation, or itching often intensifies. The itching and irritation, in turn, can make sexual activity uncomfortable; the odor is often a "turn off" to sex partners so foreplay, oral sex, or intercourse is avoided. BV will not heal, or disappear, on its own. There are no over-the-counter remedies available to treat BV. Therefore, a proper diagnosis and individualized treatment plan is necessary.

Diagnosis

A health-care practitioner will take a thorough medical and sexual history from a woman presenting for treatment. A health-care practitioner will ask about sex partners, use of contraceptives, including oral contraceptive pills and other methods, and hygiene practices. A physical examination, including a pelvic examination, is required. During the pelvic examination, the health-care practitioner is looking for thin, white discharge that adheres to or coats the vaginal walls. It is possible to take a sample of the vaginal fluid and use litmus paper to instantly tell if the vaginal pH is alkaline (i.e., >4.5). A swab of the vaginal discharge can be taken and sent to a laboratory for microscopic analysis. However, microscopic analysis is rarely needed to confirm BV.

A woman's health and sexual history, complaints, the presence of the characteristic vaginal odor, and the white discharge coating the vagina are often sufficient to diagnose BV. However, most health-care practitioners will perform an additional test during the exam. A health-care provider will take an additional sample of the vaginal discharge and smear it on a glass microscope slide. Several drops of 10 percent potassium hydroxide (KOH) will be added to the slide. Almost instantly, the reaction between the KOH and the G. *vaginalis* releases a strong, unique, amine, or fishy odor (called the "whiff test"). The slide dries and is examined under a microscope in the clinic or office. Clue cells or vaginal epithelial cells that have coccobacilli attached to them are readily visible and solidify a diagnosis. Most health-care practitioners will not wait for any confirmatory culture results, if taken, from a laboratory; a woman's clinical presentation and the findings from a pelvic examination are often sufficient to warrant prescribing antibiotic treatment. Some women, further, have no symptoms at all and the presence of BV is found during a routine Pap test analysis.

Treatment

BV is cured only by using antibiotics. Antibiotics will relieve a woman's symptoms and remove the signs of the infection. There are a host of options for health-care practitioners to prescribe depending on a woman's needs. Typically, antifungals like metronidazole are used. Metronidazole can be prescribed as an oral tablet that is taken twice daily for seven days or as a gel that is inserted into the vagina nightly for five days. There are other antibiotic regimens that can be used that are equally effective if a woman is unable to take metronidazole.

While on metronidazole, it is important for a woman to avoid alcohol. The combination of alcohol and metronidazole causes a reaction in the body that leads to dizziness, nausea and vomiting, and an unrelenting headache. Women should avoid alcohol, then, for the duration of time they are using metronidazole and for 24 hours after the treatment is completed. While on any prescribed treatment for BV, a woman should abstain from sex or use condoms properly and consistently. Douching should be avoided; it does not hasten the cure for BV and could, in fact, make it worse. Completing all prescribed medication will likely cure the condition.

Treating BV is especially important if a woman is pregnant. Some women have BV but may not notice, or be bothered by, any symptoms. Often during routine screening for prenatal care a woman may discover she has BV. Untreated BV can lead to preterm labor and possibly the delivery of a premature or very low birth weight baby.

Treating male sex partners is often not necessary since males do not transmit BV from woman to woman. Female sex partners, however, may need an evaluation by a health-care practitioner and possibly treatment with antibiotics since BV can be transferred between women.

Prevention

The only way to prevent BV is to abstain from sex. Since total abstinence is not a viable option for most women, using condoms helps minimize the chances of the vaginal lining coming in contact with alkaline semen or the skin of the penis. Women should avoid douching; there is no evidence to support that douching is effective. Douching only depletes the vagina of its natural, protective microorganisms and thereby increases the chances of contracting BV. Normal showering and bathing are sufficient for maintaining body hygiene and vaginal cleanliness.

BV cannot be contracted from pools, hot tubs, or toilet seats. G. *vaginalis*, however, can be transferred from woman to woman during female sex, especially where sex toys are used. Any sex toy, including vibrators or dildos, or any item that is inserted into the vagina during sex should be washed thoroughly either with warm, soapy water or according to the manufacturer's instructions. Sex toys should not be stored without proper cleaning, nor should they be used again until they have been properly cleaned.

Since a woman's body reacts to her environment, a woman should minimize stressors in her life while maintaining a healthy diet and exercise plan. Proper nutrition, then, is key to providing the body with nutrients and natural probiotic microorganisms to maintain a healthy, natural flora within the vagina. Lack of sleep, alcohol intake, lack of exercise, and a diet lacking in proper nutrients all contribute to changes in a woman's body chemistry that can ultimately change her vaginal pH and allow G. *vaginalis* to proliferate, leading to BV.

Early treatment of BV helps eradicate the infection faster. Self-treatment is not a possibility since no over-the-counter products or nutritional supplements are available to cure BV. A woman should not be embarrassed to seek a medical evaluation; the odor and discharge of BV are useful to make a diagnosis and health-care practitioners specializing in women's health are accustomed to managing these complaints. While the symptoms of BV may subside on their own, most women require prescription antibiotics to effectively treat the infection.

BV can recur. The same sex partner can continue altering a woman's vaginal pH and let G. *vaginalis* grow again. Multiple sex partners, or a new sex partner, put a woman at a greater risk for having a BV infection. Safe-sex practices with the proper and consistent use of condoms, coupled with a healthy lifestyle with a balanced diet, exercise, sleep, hygiene, and stress management remain the best defense against a BV infection.

25. What are "water warts"?

"Water warts," or molluscum contagiosum, is a viral infection of the skin and the mucous membranes. It is caused by a DNA proxivirus called the molluscum contagiosum virus (MCV). The MC virus is spread from person to person by touching affected skin, such as during sexual activity. The virus may also be spread by touching a surface that has the virus on it, such as clothing, towels, or sex toys.

There are multiple types of MC virus known. MCV-1 is the most prevalent but MCV-2 is seen usually in adults. MC can affect any area of the skin but is most common on the trunk of the body, lower abdomen, groin, and legs. While MC is highly contagious from person to person while the "water warts" are visible, most people never seek treatment for it.

Additionally, the condition may persist for up to four years if untreated, yet leave no residual or lasting effects on the body.MC, however, is more common in people with weakened immune systems.

As the MC virus is passed from one person to another, the virus invades the pores or top layer of skin (called the epidermis) and begins to multiply. As it grows, painless, often itchy bumps or pimples develop on the skin. When these bumps or pimples are squeezed, a clear, non-odorous, scant amount of fluid is released. This fluid, in turn, can cause new bumps or pimples to form, and the cycle continues. Since there is prolonged intimate body contact during sexual activity, MC is easy to transmit from person to person, hence why it is classified along with other STDs.

Signs and Symptoms

MC lesions will only appear on the skin; unlike other STDs, they do not appear on mucous membranes such as inside the penis, vagina, or rectum. The lesions, known as mollusca, are small, raised, typically white, pink, or flesh-colored with a characteristic dimple or depression in the center. There can be a single lesion or aggregates of them. They are often pearly or shiny in appearance and can be soft or firm to touch. The size of each lesion varies; they can be as tiny as a pinhead to as large as a pencil eraser. Regardless of the size, the lesions are often itchy with the itching aggravated by heat, hot showers, perspiration, or clothing.

Diagnosis

MC has a characteristic appearance unlike other lesions. Diagnosis is typically made by visually inspecting the lesions and the skin and tissues surrounding them. A health-care practitioner will take a thorough health and sexual history prior to the physical examination. There are no laboratory tests, swabs, or specimens needed to make the diagnosis. Since MC appears more often in people with weakened immune systems, a health-care practitioner may recommend additional blood tests or HIV screening.

Treatment

Most MC lesions do not need treatment unless they are in the genital area such as the tip of the penis or on or near the vagina or rectum. Because these areas are exposed repeatedly to irritants (e.g., urine, sexual activity, clothing), there is an increased risk of the lesions becoming scratched and infected. Additionally, the presence of the lesions in the genital area serves as a portal for transmission of other STDs through sex, body contact, or contact with a partner's infected body fluids. Treatment, then, is aimed at removing or minimizing the lesions.

Lesions can be removed in several ways. Physical removal of the lesions can be accomplished through cryotherapy (a targeted blast of liquid nitrogen that freezes and destroys the lesion) and curettage (scraping the lesion and a small amount of the tissue surrounding it off), or through laser therapy (a targeted beam of a laser quickly burns off the lesion). Physically removing the lesions is quick and can be done with a minimal amount of local anesthesia. The procedure itself is often painless but there is typically soreness or discomfort following the procedure as the area heals.

The lesions can also be removed by taking a prescription medication. Medication regimens vary, but they require a person to take a prescribed dose of medication for several days or weeks. While there is no pain associated with taking prescribed oral therapy, the results, unlike physical removal, may take several weeks to achieve.

There are also medicated creams or lotions that can be applied directly to the skin and the lesions themselves. With topical therapy, each individual lesion requires treatment. Treating one MC lesion treats that MC lesion only; there is no way to treat any potential MC lesions or ones that might be in the process of erupting. There are several options available for topical treatment but the most common are podophyllotoxin cream or imiquimod. Topical medications burn or fry the outer layers of the MC lesions and aid in drying the fluid that is contained within them, thereby destroying the MC virus. Topical treatment can be applied by a health-care professional or the person themselves. Often there is a stinging or burning sensation with each topical application that lessens over time with each repeated application. Blistering or scabbing may occur at the site of application and persist until the area heals. It is important for anyone using topical medication to thoroughly wash their hands prior to and immediately after applying the medication and to not use the topical medication for any other skin condition other than the MC lesions. Additionally, the topical medication should not be shared with anyone else and once the lesion is healed all remaining topical medication should be discarded.

Additional Considerations

Since the MC virus lives only on the top layer of the skin, once the layers slough and are regenerated the virus typically dies off and disappears.

Unlike other STDs caused by viruses, the MC virus does not lie dormant and flare-up from time to time (e.g., the herpes virus). However, a person can contract MC again, or repeatedly, if they come in contact with the virus another time. Unlike most other STDs, MC can be contracted by contact with clothing, towels, or items around a pool or sauna. While there are several treatment options available, a person with MC should be evaluated by a health-care practitioner who can develop an individualized treatment plan for each person. Self-treating with products found on the Internet or with home remedies is not recommended and can be harmful.

Prevention

Since the MC virus lives on the skin, maintaining good hygiene habits helps minimize the amount of MC virus found on the skin. Along with good hygiene, regular hand washing should be practiced to not only prevent spreading MC virus to other parts of the body but also remove other harmful germs that can be picked up from contact with other people or surfaces.

If one has an MC lesion, it is important not to touch, pick, squeeze, or scratch the lesion or the area surrounding it. Scratching or touching the lesion can spread the MC virus to other parts of the body or expose that area to other harmful bacteria. To minimize touching or scratching the lesion, keep the area covered with a bandage or layers of light clothing that can be easily washed prior to rewearing.

Any activities that require close skin-to-skin contact should be avoided. These include contact sports like wrestling, basketball, or football unless the lesions can be adequately covered by a bandage or clothing. Additionally, sharing of gear like helmets, gloves, or other sports items should be avoided.

When MC lesions are present, it is also important to not shave, wax, or use hair remover on areas where the lesions are present. Sharing personal items, further, such as hair brushes, towels, wrist watches, or bar soaps should be avoided. Similarly, when MC lesions are present in the genital area, sexual activity, including intercourse, should be avoided until the lesion heals. Alternatively, the proper and consistent use of condoms can help minimize the transmission of the MC virus. Sex toys or other items inserted into the vagina or rectum should not be shared unless they are thoroughly cleaned with warm soapy water and properly dried between use and partners.

26. What is chancroid?

Chancroid is an STD that is caused by a bacterium, *Haemophilus ducreyi*, or *H. ducreyi*, that is passed from person to person during sexual contact.

While the incidence of chancroid has declined significantly in the United States, it is still prevalent in other parts of the world such as the Caribbean, Africa, or Southeast Asia. Most people who are diagnosed with chancroid, then, have traveled outside the United States to areas where the infection is most common.

Chancroid is often confused with the word "chancre." A chancre is a symptom associated with a viral STD. Chancroid, in contrast, is a bacterial disease itself. However, the symptoms of early chancroid include the development of an ulcer or sore that closely resembles the chancre of primary syphilis. An important distinction is that chancroid refers to a disease, while chancre refers to an ulcer or sore that is a sign or symptoms of a disease.

H. ducreyi is only spread through sexual contact or intercourse. During sexual activity, the friction from vigorous foreplay or penetration into the vagina or rectum leads to small breaks, or micro-abrasions, on the skin surfaces of the genitals or within the mucous membranes on the inside of the penis, vagina, or rectum. *H. ducreyi* enters through these micro-abrasions. Once inside the body, a local tissue reaction occurs at the site of entry and a small, reddened pimple develops. Within five to seven days the pimple grows and begins to fill with fluid, typically pus, and becomes a pustule. Eventually the pustule begins to break down, leaving a painful ulcer that can take up to several weeks to heal.

Signs and Symptoms

Chancroid is one of the STDs whose symptoms are local: they only appear at the site where the *H. ducreyi* bacterium entered the body, and there are no systemic symptoms that would alert someone to the disease. The primary symptom, then, is the pustule or ulcer found in the genital areas. Men typically notice one pustule or ulcer on the tip or head of the penis, under the foreskin if uncircumcised, on the shaft of the penis, on the scrotum, or surrounding the rectum. Women, conversely, may have several pustules or ulcers inside the vagina or at its opening, on the labia, or around or within the rectum.

The pustules often go undetected and progress to ulcers within a week. The ulcer is typically painful, especially when touched or rubbed by toilet paper, a towel, or by underwear or clothing. Urine passing over the ulcer or coming in contact with it often makes the pain intensify or cause a burning sensation. Because of its location in the genital area, urination or sexual contact or activity is often painful.

The ulcer itself can vary in size and appearance. Typically, the ulcer is about 1/8 to 2 inches in diameter (3 to 50 mm) with very well-defined borders. Those borders, however, may be irregular or jagged, so the ulcer is never a perfect circle or oval. The ulcer is usually covered with a gray or yellow material that bleeds easily when touched or scraped. The ulcer, then, is a crater. It is not possible to pop or squeeze the ulcer, and often the ulcer and its immediate surrounding tissues are tender or painful to touch. Repeatedly touching the ulcer, further, can contaminate the area with other bacteria that can cause a secondary skin infection.

If chancroid is left untreated, the *H. ducreyi* bacterium proliferates and begins to invade the tissues surrounding the ulcer. When this occurs, the lymph nodes in the inguinal area (i.e., the groin area, or the area in the fold between the hip and the genital area) begin to enlarge, harden, and become tender or painful. If treatment is further delayed, the enlarged lymph nodes can erupt through the skin and develop into a draining abscess. Early diagnosis and treatment, then, is essential.

Diagnosis

An evaluation by a health-care practitioner is necessary to correctly diagnose chancroid. The health-care practitioner will take a thorough health history, sexual history, and perform a physical examination. The physical examination will require an inspection of the genital areas, including the rectum, and often a pelvic examination for women with a speculum inserted into the vagina to allow better visualization of the inner vaginal walls and the cervix. If an ulcer is identified, a swab of the area is taken and sent to a laboratory to identify under a microscope if the *H. ducreyi* bacterium is present. Because the ulcer associated with chancroid can mimic other diseases, the health-care practitioner may also perform blood tests for syphilis. Since chancroid and syphilis are associated with a higher incidence of HIV, a health-care practitioner will likely counsel, and recommend testing for, HIV.

While chancroid and syphilis are different diseases, both diseases share the development of an ulcer somewhere in the genital area as a common symptom. Because the ulcer looks similar in both diseases, a health-care practitioner cannot make a definitive diagnosis from inspection alone. Therefore, additional laboratory testing is needed (e.g., swabs taken from the ulcer for microscopic analysis and blood tests). What will distinguish chancroid from syphilis is the identification of the *H. ducreyi* bacterium. Since both chancroid and syphilis are caused by bacteria, treatment with antibiotics can successfully eradicate both diseases. The treatment regimens, however, differ.

Treatment

Chancroid, if found early, is highly responsive to specific antibiotics. Typically, a single dose of antibiotics, either as a single pill (e.g., azithromycin) or several tablets taken all at once, or a single injection of antibiotics (e.g., ceftriaxone) into a muscle is sufficient to kill off *H. ducreyi*. Another option is a prescription for erythromycin tablets taken for several days. Treating the sexual partners of a person diagnosed with chancroid may also be required with similar antibiotic therapy.

If the *H. ducreyi* bacterium has infiltrated the surrounding tissues and causes the lymph nodes in that area to enlarge, additional antibiotics are often required. Multiple antibiotics are prescribed not only to kill off *H. ducreyi* but also kill off the microorganisms that may be causing a secondary skin infection or the enlargement of the adjacent lymph nodes. If the adjacent lymph nodes are severely swollen or abscessed, they may need to be incised and drained and treated with additional antibiotics.

Chancroid is typically responsive to antibiotics and the disease, overall, can be cured. There are usually no adverse side effects from having chancroid or from its treatment. The biggest risk of having chancroid, then, is the possibility of a secondary infection developing around the site of the ulcer, or the potential for lymph nodes to enlarge and abscess. While having chancroid poses no lifelong consequences to the person diagnosed with it, prevention of chancroid, like other STDs, remains a priority.

Additional Considerations

Having a chancroid sore or ulcer increases one's risk of contracting HIV or other STDs, like syphilis. It is important, then, to have regular health screenings and evaluations by a health-care practitioner. A health-care practitioner can develop an individualized plan for routine screening tests for HIV and other STDs.

Prevention

Like the other STDs, abstinence from sexual activity is the only definitive way to prevent chancroid. Since the bacterium that causes chancroid is passed easily during sexual activity, one of the practical ways to prevent spreading chancroid is through the proper and consistent use of condoms. Condoms serve as a barrier to spreading the bacterium from partner to partner. Therefore, using female condoms or latex condoms for vaginal or anal sex can be effective. Since small abrasions or breaks in the skin of the genital area can happen during foreplay or vigorous sexual activity, the use of lubricants can help minimize friction and aid in preserving the integrity of the skin and mucous membranes in the genital area.

If one suspects a pimple, pustule, or ulcer is forming in the genital area, it is important to avoid touching, probing, or scratching that area. Touching the area introduces additional harmful bacteria into the ulcer and the tissue surrounding it but also poses the potential to spread the *H. ducreyi* bacterium to other genital areas or parts of the body. Thorough and consistent hand washing with soap and water, then, helps minimize the amounts of harmful bacteria on the hands that could potentially cause a secondary infection in and around the ulcer.

27. What is HPV?

Human papillomavirus, or HPV, is the most common viral sexually transmitted disease currently. It has become so common that the CDC estimates that nearly all sexually active men and women will be infected with HPV at some point in their lives. HPV is actually a group of more than 150 related viruses, with each virus given a number called its HPV type. Within this large group of viruses, there are about 40 specific HPV types that are known to infect the male and female genital area. While most people with HPV will never develop any specific disease, a significant majority of people with HPV will develop conditions such as genital warts or potentially lethal cancers of the genital area.

HPV is transmitted easily through intimate skin-to-skin contact. Oral, vaginal, and anal sex, then, provides the most common pathway for transmitting HPV. Like many other STDs, a person can be infected with HPV and not know they have it. Further, a person does not need to have any active disease or symptoms to pass the HPV to an uninfected person. The virus can remain within a person's body for years before any disease or symptoms develop.

Each strain of HPV causes a different disease or condition in the body. For example, HPV 6 and HPV 11 typically cause genital warts. Other strains of HPV have been implicated in several forms of genital cancer. For example, HPV 16 and HPV 18 cause about 70 percent of cervical cancers. Other high risk strains, such as HPV 31, 33, 45, 52, and 58, have been identified as causes of cancer in the vulva, vagina, penis, or anus. They can also cause cancer in the back of the throat, the base of the tongue, and the tonsils. Cancers, however, can take years, and possibly decades, to develop after a person becomes infected with HPV.

Signs and Symptoms

Because there are so many different strains of HPV, signs and symptoms, then, depend on how the disease manifests itself in the body. For example, a person who is infected with HPV 6 or HPV 11 will display symptoms of genital warts such as small bumps, or a group of bumps, in the genital area that can be small or large, raised or flat, or resemble small pieces of cauliflower. Cancers caused by HPV, however, do not have signs or symptoms until the cancers are advanced, serious, and the most difficult to treat. Screening tests and early diagnosis, then, are essential for identifying early signs of disease to allow treatment to begin before the disease reaches advanced stages.

Diagnosis

The first step to diagnosing HPV is to have a complete health and physical examination completed by a health-care practitioner. The genital areas will be examined closely, often with a light or magnifier to make inspecting the areas easier. For women, a pelvic examination is often included so the health-care practitioner can see the cervix and inner walls of the vagina. During the pelvic examination, a Pap test of the cervix is also obtained. The Pap test is a gentle swabbing, brushing, or scraping of the cervix to obtain cells from its surface. Aside from being able to detect the presence of HPV, the Pap test may also identify changes to the other cells or precancerous changes to the cervix that would warrant further evaluation or more frequent screening. For visible lesions, the health-care practitioner is able to swab the area and obtain a viral culture to diagnose the presence, and specific strain of, HPV. If a woman is pregnant, it is imperative to have a full examination by a health-care practitioner. HPV is transmissible to a baby from its mother during pregnancy. Therefore, proper diagnosis, and treatment, is essential prior to becoming pregnant or immediately after a woman discovers she is pregnant.

Cervical cancers can be detected, then, with routine cervical cancer screening through the Pap test. Specific to the cervix, the Pap test can identify abnormal cells on the cervix so they can be removed before cancer develops. An HPV DNA test is available that can be used in conjunction with a Pap test to identify certain HPV types on a woman's cervix. If a woman has received the HPV vaccine, she still requires regular cervical cancer screening because the vaccine, while effective, does not protect a woman against all cervical cancers.

While HPV can also cause cancers of the anus, penis, or the back of the throat, there is currently no routinely recommended screening tests to identify these types of cancers early. Screening test have been developed and refined, but more information is needed to determine their overall effectiveness.

Treatment

There is no treatment that will destroy HPV. However, treatments are available for the individual conditions HPV causes.

- Genital warts—Only visible warts can be treated. The type of treatment depends upon the location of the warts, how many warts there are, and what the warts look like. Treatment, then, is aimed at getting rid of the visible warts and lowering the amount of virus present. While there are several types of treatment available, such as medicated creams, freezing with liquid nitrogen, burning the warts off with electrocautery, surgical removal or removal with a laser, successful treatment does not guarantee the warts will not recur. Additionally, a combination of treatments is often the most effective. At present, there is no over-the-counter treatment one can buy to treat genital warts. Further, wart remover creams, gels, or pads that one would purchase over the counter and use on the hands or other parts of the body do not work on genital warts and should not be used. While genital warts will eventually go away if untreated, they tend to enlarge and become increasingly ugly or distressing to look at. Treating the warts, then, greatly reduces the risk of passing them on to another person and speeds the healing of the warts.
- Abnormal cervical cells—While abnormal cervical cells often become normal over time, they sometimes turn into cancer. Treatment for these abnormal cells depends on the severity of the cell changes, the woman's age and past medical history, and other test results. Minimally invasive methods and procedures are available for removing layers of abnormal cells from the cervix.
- Cervical cancer—is most treatable when it is diagnosed and treated early. Problems found can usually be treated depending on several factors including a woman's age, health status, medical history, and the severity of the cancer found. While routine screening helps identify cancers earlier, preventing cancers is more effective than treating them.

Prevention

The only definitive way to prevent contracting any of the various strains of HPV is to abstain from sexual activity. Since abstinence is not a common or preferred option in modern times, barrier methods such as condoms help lower the risk of spreading HPV. Condoms, however, only cover a specific surface area of the penis or vagina. HPV is spread from skin-to-skin contact, so the genital region can still come in contact with HPV from touching the thighs, scrotum, or other genital skin of an infected person. With genital warts, further, most people often are unaware that they are infected and fail to use condoms properly and consistently to minimize any potential transmission of HPV.

A vaccine was developed that can protect women from conditions that develop because of HPV. Specifically, girls immunized at a young age are potentially protected from lethal cancers later in life. By vaccinating girls, and boys, between the ages of 9 to 26, it is hoped that protection against HPV will begin before the onset of sexual activity and remain with them through adulthood. In contrast, receiving the vaccine later in adulthood has demonstrated little to no efficacy against cervical cancers or genital warts. The HPV vaccine (known as Cervarix, Gardasil and now Gardasil-9) not only protects against the various strains of HPV that cause cervical cancers but also protects against strains of HPV that cause 90 percent of genital warts. The vaccine, administered as a series of three injections spaced out over a six-month period, is not without controversy. While scientific evidence continues to demonstrate the efficacy of the vaccine, parents are reluctant to vaccinate their children in anticipation of a sexually transmitted disease or cancer that they may or may not get. Pediatricians, further, are divided among their professional organizations; opinions about whether or not to vaccinate are inconsistent. Despite the controversies surrounding the HPV vaccine, the scientific data regarding the HPV vaccine is compelling and encouraging regarding cervical cancers and genital warts. Careful analysis, then, of the risks and benefits of the vaccine should be explored and weighed by parents and health-care practitioners alike.

28. What is pelvic inflammatory disease?

Pelvic inflammatory disease, or PID, is a serious medical condition for women that are often the result of untreated, or improperly treated, sexually transmitted diseases. Women develop PID when certain microorganisms, such as the bacteria that cause chlamydia or gonorrhea, migrate upward from the woman's vagina or cervix and infect the organs of the upper genital tract such as the uterus, fallopian tubes, or ovaries. While the bacteria that cause chlamydia and gonorrhea are the most common causes of PID, the vagina can contain a variety of other microorganisms that can proliferate inappropriately, for example, when a woman has bacterial vaginosis, and cause PID. Without proper treatment, PID can permanently damage a woman's reproductive organs, leading to infertility.

Signs and Symptoms

Women can exhibit a variety of signs and symptoms with PID. When symptoms are present, they can mimic those that are common with urinary or gastrointestinal conditions. The most common symptoms of PID, then, include fever, lower abdominal pain, painful urination or intercourse, irregular vaginal bleeding, or an increased vaginal discharge. The abdominal pain or pelvic discomfort, however, is what typically drives women to see an evaluation by a health-care practitioner.

Diagnosis

Diagnosis of PID requires a thorough medical history review and physical examination by a health-care practitioner. The physical examination will also include a pelvic examination. During the pelvic examination, the health-care practitioner will look at any vaginal discharge and take cultures from the vagina or cervix to hopefully identify chlamydia, gonorrhea, or other STDs. Part of the pelvic examination includes a bimanual examination. With a bimanual examination, the health-care practitioner gently inserts the index and middle fingers into the vagina to stabilize and palpate the cervix, while using the other hand to gently palpate the lower abdomen which permits him or her to feel the body of the uterus, the fallopian tubes, ovaries, and other structures. With PID, the lower abdomen and the area surrounding the uterus and ovaries is tender to touch and uncomfortable for the woman. Moving or touching the cervix, further, causes additional pain and discomfort. When the physical and pelvic examinations are complete, the health-care practitioner may order laboratory blood tests to look for elevated white blood cell counts or other values that would indicate infection or inflammation. The woman's presenting symptoms, and the findings of the physical and pelvic examinations, however, are often sufficient enough to begin treatment.

Treatment

PID is treatable with antibiotics. Typically, broad spectrum antibiotics, or antibiotics that are powerful enough to kill several microorganisms at one time, are used. These antibiotics can be given orally; often the symptoms a woman is experiencing warrant hospitalization where antibiotics and other drugs to manage the symptoms can be given intravenously. While antibiotics can cure the immediate infection and inflammation, they cannot reverse any scarring or damage to a woman's reproductive organs.

In most cases, the male sex partners of a woman diagnosed with PID will require treatment with antibiotics, even if he exhibits no signs or symptoms of an STD. Since chlamydia and gonorrhea are the most common STDs leading to PID, treating male partners not only cures any potential disease but also prevents the male partner from reinfecting a woman once her course of PID treatment is completed.

Additional Considerations

Once treatment for PID has begun, the symptoms respond quickly and go away before PID is fully cured. Therefore, it is important for a woman to complete the entire course of the prescribed antibiotic regimen to ensure the PID is fully treated. Without complete treatment, the fallopian tubes can become scarred and predispose a woman to ectopic pregnancies in the future. Similarly, the scar tissue that can form in the pelvis from the widespread inflammation of PID may lead to chronic pelvic pain and discomfort. Improperly treated PID not only damages a woman's reproductive organs but also causes complications that can be life-threatening. Some of these complications include abscess formation of infected material around the ovaries, fallopian tubes, or both. Systemic sepsis, further, is a possibility if the infection becomes widespread and invades other organs throughout the body.

Prevention

The best way to prevent PID is to avoid opportunities to contract an STD such as chlamydia or gonorrhea. Therefore, the proper and consistent use of condoms is the most effective way to prevent the transmission of the various microorganisms that can cause STDs. Regular screening including HIV testing, then, for sexually active women allows for early diagnosis and treatment of STDs to prevent their evolution into PID. Lastly, younger women should explore vaccination for human papillomavirus (HPV); women of all ages should explore vaccination to prevent Hepatitis B.

29. What is mucopurulent cervicitis?

Mucopurulent cervicitis, or MPC, is an infection of the cervix, or opening of the uterus, that is usually the result of a woman having an STD such as chlamydia. Unprotected vaginal or anal sex, then, is the primary way microorganisms that cause STDs are transmitted to a woman that contribute to the development of an STD. Typically the bacteria that cause chlamydia, or other microorganisms that cause other STDs, multiply in the vagina and ascend into the cervix. Microorganisms can live in the cervix indefinitely but can multiply and cause an infection. When the infection occurs, the cervix inflames and a heavy vaginal discharge occurs, often accompanied by pain or discomfort with sexual activity, or irregular vaginal bleeding. Left untreated, MPC can lead to PID. Therefore, recognizing MPC early, and implementing treatment, is essential.

Signs and Symptoms

Many women are unaware they have an STD such as chlamydia or gonorrhea; by the time the symptoms, if any, are noticed, the microorganisms may have been thriving and multiplying in the vagina, or the cervix, for some time. The characteristic symptom of MPC is a thick, copious, vaginal discharge that is often creamy, white to light yellow in color, and without a strong odor. Women often notice the discharge after sex and may find small pools of discharge on their underwear or on panty liners or sanitary pads. The discharge may irritate the vaginal opening and cause itching. Irregular vaginal bleeding or spotting is common; often the spotting is light red to pink without any pain or cramping. Pain or discomfort occurs during or after sexual activity. The discharge or spotting, further, does not diminish with bathing or rest. It is often the combination of symptoms, then, that leads a woman to seek an evaluation by a health-care practitioner.

Diagnosis

A health-care practitioner will review a woman's complete medical and sexual history and perform a physical examination. The physical examination will also include a pelvic examination. With a speculum gently inserted into the vagina, a health-care practitioner can visualize and inspect the cervix. The health-care practitioner will often see an inflamed or irritated cervix that may be covered or surrounded by thick discharge. If the health-care practitioner takes a cotton-tipped applicator and wipes away, or takes a specimen of, the discharge, the cervix often bleeds easily. While the discharge and easy friability of the cervix are often sufficient to lead the health-care practitioner to diagnose MPC, specimens may also be taken to test for the presence of chlamydia and/or gonorrhea. However, the vagina and cervix are often full of multiple microorganisms once the symptoms of MPC are noticeable; isolating the specific bacteria that cause chlamydia and gonorrhea can be difficult. Therefore, health-care practitioners will often initiate treatment based on a woman's presenting symptoms and the findings of the physical and pelvic examinations.

Treatment

Since chlamydia and gonorrhea are often the cause of MPC, the health-care practitioner will implement antibiotic therapy to kill the bacteria that cause both. Typically, the treatment for both chlamydia and gonorrhea is sufficient to eradicate the MPC also. Antibiotics, given as a single dose in an oral tablet or tablets, are inexpensive and effective. Often health-care practitioners will give a combination of drugs, including broad spectrum antibiotics that can successfully kill off a variety of harmful microorganisms. Male sex partners, then, should be tested and treated also to not only prevent STDs from occurring but also prevent reinfecting a woman with an STD, or spreading an STD to others. Symptoms, then, will subside gradually and it could take a week for the antibiotics to eradicate MPC completely. The full course of antibiotics should be completed. If symptoms are not relieved, or recur, within three to four weeks, a woman should be reevaluated by a health-care practitioner.

Additional Considerations

While a woman is undergoing treatment with antibiotics for MPC, she should abstain from sexual activity to minimize any discomfort sex may cause and decrease vaginal bleeding or irritation to the cervix. If sexual activity is going to occur, condoms should be used for all vaginal or anal sex for at least 7 to 10 days following the completion of antibiotic therapy.

Prevention

Since MPC is caused by other STDs, avoiding opportunities to contract STDs like chlamydia or gonorrhea is essential. The proper and consistent use of condoms is the most effective way to prevent the transmission of the various microorganisms that cause STDs. Regular screening including HIV testing, then, for sexually active women allows for early diagnosis and treatment of STDs to prevent their evolution into PID. Lastly, younger women should explore vaccination for human papillomavirus (HPV); women of all ages should explore vaccination to prevent Hepatitis B.

30. What is lymphogranuloma venereum?

Lymphogranuloma venereum (LGV) is one of the less common STDs. Though more common in certain areas of Africa, Southeast Asia, India, the Caribbean, and South America, the increased industrialization in those areas, along with increased tourism and out-migration, have all led to outbreaks of LGV in North America, Europe, and the United Kingdom.

LGV is another type of disease that, similar to genital herpes or syphilis, causes the formation of an ulcer in the genital area. The bacterium that causes LGV is a serotype, or an invasive variation of the same microorganism that causes chlamydia, *Chlamydia trachomatis* (*C. trachomatis*). The bacterium gains entrance into the body through a break in the skin or, more typically, through contact with the mucous membranes of the mouth, vagina, or rectum. The bacterium then travels from the point of entry through the lymphatic channels in the body. As it passes through the lymph nodes, it attaches to the cells the body uses to destroy invading microorganisms. Instead of being destroyed, the bacterium multiplies.

Signs and Symptoms

The signs and symptoms of LGV depend on where the site of entry for the bacterium is located. A sore, or an ulcer, develops at the site of entry. If the site of entry is the lining on the inside, or tip of the penis, or within or around the vagina, the sore can be reddened with a hard, yellow crusted surface over it, or a pale crater. The area is often painful, especially to contact with clothing or drops of urine. A person typically develops enlarged, swollen, tender lymph nodes or infected abscesses within the inguinal area (the area or channel between the hips and the pubic bone). Once exposed, a person may develop these symptoms anywhere from three days to one month after exposure.

Similarly, if the site of entry is the rectum, the sore or ulcer develops either at the anal opening or within the rectum itself. Bowel movements become painful. There is often burning, soreness, or itching at the site, and the area becomes tender to touch especially with sitting or wiping after a bowel movement. As the ulcer worsens, there is often increased swelling of the anus, rectum, or lower colon, leading to fevers and increased discomfort. Though rare, LGV lesions can occur also in the neck or the throat if exposure to the bacterium occurred through the mucous membranes of the mouth.

Like other STDs, LGV occurs in stages. In the primary stage, a painless genital sore or ulcer develops at the site of the bacterium's entry, typically 3–12 days after exposure. Women rarely notice any symptoms; the lesions are painless and usually located inside the vagina or at the vaginal opening where they are not readily seen. Men may notice symptoms due to irritation of the lesion by a stream of urine. Often the lesions for men are at the opening of the penis, or down inside the first two-thirds of the penis shaft, so they, too, are difficult to see. The primary stage, however, heals within a few days with many people never realizing they were infected.

The secondary stage can occur 10–30 days after the primary stage but may begin up to six months later. By this time, the bacterium has spread to the lymph nodes through the lymphatic system. The most frequent presenting symptom in the secondary stage is the enlarged, tender, lymph nodes in either the groin or inguinal area. For men, there may also be tenderness along the under surface of the penis or along the outer rim of the scrotum or testicles. For women, the symptoms of enlarged lymph nodes are present but they also complain of tenderness along the outer vagina or pubic area. If the site for the bacterium entry is the rectum from anal sex, both men and women may complain of pain at the anal opening or tenderness to the area surrounding it. Additionally, both men and women may report a feeling of pressure or fullness in the rectum despite having had recent bowel movements, increased sharp pain with each bowel movement, or a mucous-like discharge. Diarrhea, gas, and cramping are also common.

Women may experience symptoms during the secondary stage that mimics other gynecologic conditions. Women often report pain in the lower abdomen with tenderness to the abdominal area that worsens when the area is touched, poked, or examined by a health-care professional. With this abdominal pain, women often complain of fevers, decreased appetite, and an overall feeling of being run down or sick.

As the disease progresses, the lymph nodes in the groin continue to enlarge into painful, irregular-shaped tender masses called buboes. There is limited space for these buboes to grow; as a result, they adhere to the skin that is overlying them. Eventually, the skin loses its supply of blood and proteins so the area breaks down, cracks, and a crater forms. Pus can typically drain from these areas. However, the buboes keep growing and often cause abscesses (a collection of infectious material) or tracts (called fistulas) to form within the tissue surrounding the buboes. Bacteria, then, can spread through the fistulas and make the infection more widespread. If healing occurs without proper treatment, the area becomes dense and hardened, like a scar. These areas, then, can block the flow of lymph fluid leading to chronic swelling, pain, and discoloration of the thighs, groin, and lower legs.

Diagnosis

Typically, the swollen, painful lymph nodes are what drive people to seek medical attention. Because the swollen lymph nodes are also symptoms of other conditions, other diseases or illnesses get ruled out first before LGV is considered. If genital lesions are present, or the swollen node can be aspirated for a sample of fluid within it, cultures can be sent to a laboratory to identify if *C. trachomatis* is present. Blood tests are also available but are not very sensitive or confirmatory for LGV. Once all other diseases, then, are ruled out, LGV can be confirmed.

Treatment

LGV is caused by a bacterium, so treatment options are available. Most health-care practitioners will initiate treatment for LGV if the suspicion for the disease is high, even before other conditions have been ruled out. The earlier treatment is initiated, cure can occur and long-term damage avoided. Antibiotic therapy, often, in the form of pills taken twice daily for three weeks is the treatment of choice. Drugs such as doxycycline, erythromycin, or azithromycin are used. Often a secondary infection of the skin or the surrounding tissue occurs because of the spread of infectious material in and around the buboes. These secondary infections, then, can complicate treatment and make curing LGV prolonged.

If the buboes are too large, and the skin covering the area is not broken or dying, the health-care practitioner may opt to drain some or all of the fluid in and around the buboes in order to collapse them and expedite healing. Manipulating the buboes, however, does not change any long-term scarring or discoloration to the involved tissue once healing occurs. Similarly, people being treated for LGV are advised to take their antibiotics as ordered and to complete the course of therapy. Follow-up is required to determine if the treatment was effective or if an additional course of treatment is needed.

Additional Considerations

People diagnosed with LGV should also be tested for other STDs, especially gonorrhea, syphilis, and HIV. Testing positive for other STDs does not alter a treatment plan for LGV; however, additional treatment regimens may be indicated along with follow-up cultures or laboratory blood tests, depending on the diagnosis, to confirm each condition was cured.

Sex partners of people diagnosed with LGV require a medical evaluation also. Sex partners who have contact with someone diagnosed with LGV within 60 days of the onset of symptoms should be examined and tested for penile, vaginal, or rectal chlamydia infections. If no lesions are found, and before any cultures or laboratory blood tests are resulted, sex partners will often be treated presumptively with an antibiotic regimen to halt the disease progression and minimize any complications that may arise. Presumptive treatment for sex partners, unlike the person being treated for active LGV disease, is of a shorter duration and typically ranges from a one-time oral dose of antibiotic medication to a course of antibiotic pills taken orally twice each day for a week.

Prevention

Prevention of LGV is possible through the proper and consistent use of condoms for oral, vaginal, and anal sex. Like many other STDs, a person is often unaware they have LGV. Transmission, then, can occur without warning signs. Condoms provide a barrier to protect oral, vaginal, and anal surfaces from being exposed to the body fluids of an infected person. Additionally, a healthy body is more resilient to fighting off infections, and less likely to have tissues break down due to stress or vigorous sexual activity. Therefore, proper nutrition and exercise are essential to maintaining overall good health.

31. Is a yeast infection an STD?

Yeast infections are not STDs. However, sexual activity, spermicidal creams, and lubricants can cause changes in the pH of the vagina and allow yeast to grow and proliferate leading to a vaginal yeast infection. It is estimated that three out of four women may experience a vaginal yeast infection at some point in their lives regardless of age.

Yeast infections are caused by a naturally occurring fungus called Candida albicans (*C. albicans*). *C.albicans* lives in moist areas of the body such as the mouth, skin folds, groin, and vagina. Certain conditions, then, can alter the vagina's pH and allow *C. albicans* to proliferate, thereby increasing the risk of contracting a yeast infection. These conditions include: taking medications such as antibiotics or steroids, having uncontrolled diabetes, experiencing hormonal changes such as those common with pregnancy or with the use of birth control pills, using bubble baths, wearing tight-fitting clothes, using feminine hygiene products such as douches or regularly using spermicidal gels or lubricants during sex. Sex alone does not give a woman a yeast infection; *C. albicans* is not transmitted from one person to another like other STDs. However, the skin of the penis carries its own colony of normal microorganisms that, when introduced into the vagina during sex, could alter a woman's own normal vaginal flora of microorganisms, thereby allowing *C. albicans* to overgrow and lead to a vaginal yeast infection.

Signs and Symptoms

The most common symptom of a vaginal yeast infection is intense itching inside the vagina or at the vaginal opening. Vaginal discharge is common and many women will notice white or pale gray colored discharge at the vagina opening or on their underwear or sanitary pads. The discharge is often thick and may resemble the consistency of cottage cheese. The discharge typically has no odor. With the intense itching, the vagina or the vaginal opening often becomes reddened and irritated from the both the presence of the irritating discharge and the scratching used to relieve the itching. Since the vaginal area is inflamed and irritated, there is often pain or burning with urination. Similarly, sexual activity is equally as painful. Vaginal soreness will intensify with prolonged sitting, walking, or other physical activity. The symptoms, therefore, are often what compel a woman to seek treatment.

Diagnosis

If a woman seeks an evaluation by a health-care practitioner, a thorough medical and sexual history will be reviewed. A physical examination, including a pelvic examination, will follow. During the pelvic examination, a speculum is inserted in the vagina and gently opened to allow the health-care practitioner to inspect the vagina and the cervix. Typically, with a vaginal yeast infection, the vagina is dark pink to reddened with white discharge adhered to the vaginal walls and cervix. A sample of the discharge can be examined under a microscope to identify the presence of *C. albicans*. However, a woman's symptoms, coupled with the findings of the physical and pelvic examinations, are often sufficient for a health-care practitioner to confirm a diagnosis of a vaginal yeast infection and implement treatment.

Treatment

Since vaginal yeast infections are caused by a fungus, antifungal medications successfully eradicate the condition and help return the flora in the vagina to its natural balance. Antifungal medications come in various forms. Some medications are prescribed as a one-time dose in a single tablet (e.g., Fluconazole), while others are prescribed as creams, ointments, or suppositories that are inserted in the vagina directly, typically at night.

Over-the-counter remedies are available that effectively treat a vaginal yeast infection. Many women mistake any vaginal discharge for a yeast infection and opt to self-treat. Vaginal discharge, however, is often a symptom of other conditions and requires an evaluation by a health-care practitioner and possibly individualized antibiotic therapy. Some women, conversely, have repeated vaginal yeast infections and are familiar with its symptoms and presentation; over-the-counter remedies provide a viable option for relief of symptoms and a treatment for a recurrent vaginal yeast infection.

Prevention

There are steps a woman can take to reduce her risk of, or prevent, a yeast infection. Among these include:

- Do not douche. Douching removes the normal flora of microorganisms in the vagina that protects a woman from a vaginal yeast infection.
- Avoid using scented feminine hygiene products such as bubble baths, vaginal sprays, sanitary pads, or tampons.
- Change sanitary pads, tampons, or panty liners regularly.

- Avoid wearing tight pants, jeans, underwear, or pantyhose. Tight clothing increases body heat and moisture in the genital area that can promote the overgrowth of *C. albicans*.
- Wear cotton underwear. Cotton underwear promotes dryness and minimizes body heat and moisture in the genital area.
- Change out of wet swimsuits, exercise clothing, or yoga pants as soon as possible.
- Always wipe from front to back after urinating or after a bowel movement.
- Avoid hot tubs or hot tub baths.
- Maintain blood sugar in normal ranges if diabetic.

Often women will eat yogurt, or take over-the-counter *Lactobacillus acidophilus* tablets to prevent a vaginal yeast infection. Evidence at present to support this is weak. There are various formulations of yogurt available for purchase and not all contain sufficient amounts of live, active yogurt cultures necessary to repopulate the vagina with healthy lactobacilli. Further, the active culture of lactobacillus in yogurt is broken down in the gut by digestion and may have no impact on the flora of microorganisms in the vagina. More research, then, is needed to demonstrate if eating yogurt with lactobacillus, or taking other forms of probiotics, can prevent or assist in treating vaginal yeast infections.

32. Can men get a yeast infection?

Men, too, can contract a yeast infection. Typically, the fungus *Candida albicans* (*C. albicans*) infects the tip of the penis and causes it to inflame or swell, a condition known as balanitis. If a man is uncircumcised, the foreskin covering the tip of the penis can also become inflamed (known as posthitis).

There are several causes of penile yeast, or balanitis. For example, in uncircumcised men, the foreskin may be too tight covering the tip of the penis, leading to a chronic dermatitis and damage to the foreskin, thereby providing a medium for *C. albicans* to overgrow. Similarly, men who are diabetic are equally at risk for developing a genital yeast infection. Whereas women do not contract a vaginal yeast infection from having sex with male partners, women can pass *C. albicans* on to male sex partners during sex. Following sexual activity, *C. albicans* can remain on or at the tip of the penis and begin to multiply. A man, in turn, will not pass *C. albicans* on to any other female sex partners.

Signs and Symptoms

Men may have no symptoms of a penile yeast infection. Males may notice discomfort or irritation at the tip or head of the penis, especially with urinating or ejaculating semen. Often the tip of the penis, or the foreskin if present, itches and may become reddened. The tip of the penis becomes sore and tender to touch. If uncircumcised, there may be a thickened, lumpy, malodorous discharge underneath the foreskin once it is retracted. Attempting to pull back, or retract, the foreskin may be painful and often unsuccessful.

Diagnosis

The pain and discomfort men experience is often what compels them to seek a medical evaluation. A health-care practitioner will take and review a thorough medical and sexual history, and perform a physical examination. The health-care practitioner will inspect the penis, including the tip and inside the opening, the foreskin, testicles, and lymph nodes in the groin. If there is significant discharge, the health-care practitioner may take a specimen so that it can be analyzed under a microscope in a laboratory to identify specific microorganisms. Urine or blood tests may also be indicated.

Treatment

Treatment usually begins immediately based upon the health-care practitioner's review of a man's medical and sexual history and the findings of the physical examination. Like women, antifungal medications are effective for decreasing the overgrowth of *C. albicans* and minimizing any symptoms a man is experiencing. Medication can be prescribed as a one-time dose of an antifungal medication (e.g., Fluconazole) taken orally in one tablet, or with antifungal creams applied to the tip of the penis and under the foreskin if present twice daily for several days. Sexual activity should be avoided until all symptoms subside.

Prevention

The proper and consistent use of condoms provides sufficient protection for men to avoid contact with *C. albicans* that may be present in the vagina during sexual activity. Good hygiene, however, remains the most effective way for men to avoid penile yeast infections. Each day, men should clean the genital area with warm, soapy water. If uncircumcised, the foreskin of the penis should be retracted and the area underneath it cleaned and dried thoroughly. Men may periodically use antifungal creams at the penile tip or under the foreskin to prevent a recurrent infection.

33. What are "crabs"?

Pubic lice (or more commonly called "crabs") are not a traditional illness or disease in the STD categories. It is often thought of, or referred to, as an STD because intimate sexual contact is the most common way crabs are transmitted from a person who has crabs to someone who does not. While crabs are curable once identified, often several days or weeks may pass from the time of contact and catching crabs to noticing the onset of symptoms. During that time, it is possible to infect new sex partners or to continue to pass crabs back and forth with existing partners. The pubic lice also multiply and can grow quickly in the days or weeks before it's discovered.

While sexual activity is the most common way of transmitting crabs, it is not the only way or source for acquiring the lice. Lice are common in countries with high levels of poverty and poor sanitation. Poor bodily hygiene, wearing the same clothes every day without washing them thoroughly, or sharing of clothes can also contribute to the growth of lice. Close contact, then, is all that is required for the lice, or crabs, to pass from person to person.

There are different types of lice and each is unique in appearance and what areas of the body they infest. Lice do not fly or have wings. Lice, in general, are tiny insects that live on humans and feed on blood. The lice insect bites the skin of the human host carrying it and the small amount of blood it receives from that bite is enough to sustain the insect for several days. Head lice, then, are often found in hair, typically at the back of the neck or behind the ears. Head lice adheres itself to the base of the hair and will often lay its eggs (called "nits") in the same area. Body lice, or scabies, in contrast, tend to live in or on clothing or fabrics and adheres itself to the skin anywhere on the body, burrowing into the first layers in order to feed and sustain itself. Pubic lice, or crabs, are typically found in the genital area among the pubic hair. Similarly, pubic lice can be found in chest hair, facial hair, beards and moustaches, armpit hair, eyebrows or even eyelashes. Pubic lice are rarely found on the scalp.

Pubic lice are tiny and can often be missed if the pubic area is not examined closely. Often a health-care practitioner will use a fine tooth comb to slowly separate the pubic hairs, or employ a bright examination light and magnifier to see the lice better. Pubic lice resemble tiny pieces of brown rice or dirt particles where the pubic hair meets the skin. Pubic lice have multiple legs and the insect uses them to crawl up and down the hair shaft or to firmly anchor themselves to the hair shaft. Often combing through the pubic hair, then, is the only thing that will dislodge the lice from the base of the pubic hair.

Signs, Symptom, and Diagnosis

Crabs are difficult to see with the naked eye. The most common symptom is itching. The itching becomes more severe, frequent, and persistent. The skin in the pubic region can be irritated or raw from the frequent scratching, and people may use objects that are more abrasive to scratch the area in the hope of relieving the itch. Irritated or reddened skin from scratching can make identifying the tiny insect bites from the lice difficult to visualize. Often the intensity of the itching, and the location, is sufficient for a health-care practitioner to come to a diagnosis quickly. No laboratory blood work or specific testing is required.

Treatment

Pubic lice, or crabs, will not go away on its own. There are successful treatment regimens that include the use of products one can buy over the counter in a pharmacy, or by prescription. The key to successful treatment is to complete the treatment regimen as directed while taking precautions to prevent the crabs from coming back.

Treatment involves creams, lotions, or shampoos that contain a medication that kills the crabs. There are several over-the-counter medications, (e.g., Rid or Nix) that can be used. These medications work particularly well for crabs that are found early and have not had a chance to multiply. The medications are also useful if someone thinks he or she may have been exposed to crabs and wants to take advantage of the opportunity to kill off crabs early. The over-the-counter creams, lotions, or shampoos have specific directions for use and warnings that need to be understood and followed prior to use.

Often crabs progress to the point of infestation: multiple lice insects are present with their eggs. Over-the-counter medications are not strong enough to kill the existing crabs. Prescription creams, lotions, or shampoos are available that work well to rapidly, and effectively, kill off the crabs. At this stage, however, the skin in the genital area is highly irritated, or raw, from scratching or maybe infected. The itching is intense also. In addition to medications to kill the crabs, the health-care practitioner may also provide medication to calm or stop the itching (such as antihistamines) and allow the skin to heal. Antibiotics, either in pill form or in a cream, do nothing to kill the crabs but can be useful to heal the skin in the genital region that may be infected from scratching. Steroid creams or calamine lotion are another option for the health-care practitioner to prescribe to decrease the local skin discomfort or itching.

Prevention

The best way to prevent crabs is to practice regular hygiene such as showering or bathing. Soaps and shampoos strip body hair of its layers of oils that the crabs cling to. It is not necessary to take extra hot or long showers or baths. In fact, bathing or showering in water that is too hot can damage the skin overall by promoting dryness and cracking. Regular shower gel soaps are sufficient for hygiene; bar soap, however, can trap crabs and spread it to other people who may share that bar of soap.

Regardless of the color, thickness, or amount of pubic hair, crabs can adhere to any hair shaft and multiply. Shaving and trimming pubic hair has become popular. Shaving can prevent crabs; without the coarse pubic hair, the crabs have nothing to cling to. Shaving does not, however, cure crabs. Even after shaving off the pubic hair, a person still needs to complete a regimen of medicated creams, lotions, or shampoos in order to kill the crabs that may be lingering, or adhered to the base of the hair, or stubble, that was not removed by shaving. What becomes problematic is that crabs cling to other body hairs, so if one is going to shave off their pubic hair they also need to consider removing the hair from their chest, abdomen, back, and legs. Trimming, or clipping, hair, regardless of how short the hair is cut to, still leaves a base of hair that the crab can cling to. Waxing hair is similar to shaving; it is only effective if all the hair is removed.

If a person is diagnosed and treated for crabs, he or she needs to not only kill the crabs that are on his or her body but also kill any crabs that might be alive on his or her clothing or in his or her home. It is recommended that all articles of clothing, including underwear, all bed sheets and blankets, be washed in very hot water and with bleach if possible. Drying the articles of clothing and bed sheets in a hot dryer is also recommended. Further, all sex partners, regardless of whether they have symptoms of crabs or not, should do the same. Sprays or disinfectant cleaners used to clean a house or household surfaces do not kill the crabs. High heat and soapy water, then, work best. Fabrics on furniture are often safe, and typically do not provide a medium for crabs to grow on.

Sexual activity should be avoided until all the symptoms disappear and the treatment regimen is completed. Condoms or other barrier methods, birth control pills, spermicidal creams or any other form of contraception do not prevent crabs. However, basic hygiene practices, coupled with open discussions with any and all sex partners about actual or potential exposure to crabs can greatly reduce its transmission. No one needs to be embarrassed about seeking help for crabs or for having any of its symptoms evaluated. Additionally, one should not hesitate, or be embarrassed, to purchase any over-the-counter product or have prescriptions filled. Not treating crabs, however, poses additional health risks for a condition that can be easily eradicated with the proper treatment and precautions.

34. What are scabies?

Scabies differ from crabs. Where crabs are lice insects that cling to the coarse body hair typical in the pubic or genital region, scabies are tiny lice insects or mites that bite into the skin and burrow under the skin's upper layers. As they burrow, the scabies lay their eggs and, when hatched, they, too, burrow under the skin and continue to mature and eventually lay eggs. Like crabs, scabies is easily transmitted through intimate, prolonged, skin-to-skin contact such as during sexual activity. Also similar to crabs, the symptoms of scabies take several days, or up to four to six weeks, to appear, with intense itching the primary complaint. Unlike crabs, which tend to focus primarily in the pubic or genital area, scabies can bite and burrow anywhere on the body. Until the scabies bite and burrow into the skin, like crabs they can linger on clothing, bedding, or other surfaces or fabrics. Left untreated, scabies can spread throughout the skin rapidly. Scabies can become numerous and they reproduce rapidly. Therefore, scabies live on skin surfaces, clothing, and fabrics making them easy to transmit from person to person.

Scabies have a long life span. Once scabies have mated, the female remains fertile the rest of her life. As such, she deposits new eggs, or larvae, as she continues to burrow under the skin about two to three days. Those eggs, in turn, hatch in about 48 hours and will continue to burrow into the skin. Scabies, in turn, mature quickly and are able to reproduce. Hence, in a relatively short time scabies are reproducing and multiplying in numbers, leading to an infestation. Fewer than 10–15 mites, further, are all that is needed to create an infestation in an otherwise healthy person.

Signs and Symptoms

Since scabies are microscopic and difficult to see readily, there is no way to tell if a sex partner has been exposed to, or has been bitten by, scabies. When a person is infected for the first time, symptoms can take several days or two to six weeks to appear. During this time, a person infected with scabies is capable of transmitting them to other people even before the onset of symptoms.

The most common symptoms of scabies are intense itching and a streaky, red rash. As the scabies burrow and multiply, they cast off proteins and feces that cause a localized reaction to human skin. That reaction causes the intense itching while the burrowing track or tunnel the scabies are making appears as a slightly reddened, raised, itching, crooked line. The itching is characteristically worse at night but can be intense at any time of day or after exposure to a hot shower or bath, or after periods of intense sweating or exercise. A pimple-like rash is common. The rash can appear anywhere on the body, but the most common sites are between the fingers, at the wrist and elbow, the armpits, the breasts or nipple area for both sexes, the shoulder blades, waist, abdomen, buttocks, or penis. Scabies rarely infects the head, neck, face, palms of the hands, or soles of the feet. Because the itching can be intense, repeated scratching can cause breaks in the skin surfaces where bacteria from fingernails or other abrasive objects used to scratch and relieve the itch can enter the skin. When this occurs, the skin surrounding the itch becomes reddened, hot or warm to the touch, tender, or hardened as a secondary skin infection overtakes the area.

Diagnosis

Diagnosis of scabies is usually made based upon the appearance and distribution of the rash on the skin and by identifying the scabies' burrowing patterns with the streaking, crooked linear marks on the skin radiating from or at the areas of itching. If possible, skin scraping is done in an attempt to identify the scabies, their eggs, or fecal matter (called scybala) under a microscope. However, a person can still be infested with mites even if no mites, eggs, or fecal matter can be identified. Treatment can be started based on physical examination by a health-care practitioner and the history of the symptoms alone.

Treatment

Treatment is aimed at killing off the scabies and their offspring while eliminating the itching and potential for a secondary skin infection that can result from the persistent scratching. Products used to treat scabies are called "scabicides" because they kill scabies, their eggs, or both. Unlike crabs, there is no over-the-counter products one can purchase in a retail drug store or pharmacy to treat scabies. All treatment, then, is available only through a prescription from a health-care practitioner for medicated lotions, creams, or shampoos.

The scabicide is applied to the entire body, from the neck down to the feet and toes. The scabicide should be applied to a clean body and left on for a specified amount of time according to the manufacturer's instructions. Clean clothing should be worn after the specified amount of time has passed after the application of the scabicide. Usually one to two treatments with a scabicide applied correctly is sufficient to kill scabies and their eggs. Itching is likely to persist after the first treatment and may persist for up to several weeks, even if all the scabies and their eggs are killed off. If itching persists for more than two to four weeks after the treatment, or if new burrows or a pimple-like rash persists, additional rounds of treatment may be indicated. A health-care professional may prescribe additional oral medications to lessen the itching (such as antihistamines) or antibiotic pills to treat any secondary skin infection if present.

Treatment for scabies needs to be given not only to the infested person but also to their household members and sex partners, especially if there was prolonged skin-to-skin contact with the infested person. Both sexual and close personal contacts who have had direct, prolonged, skin-to-skin contact (i.e., sleeping together, cuddling) within the preceding month should be examined and treated. All persons should be treated at the same time to prevent reinfestations.

Like crabs, people with scabies and their sexual, household, and close contacts, need their bedding, clothing, and towels decontaminated. There is no commercial spray, insecticide, disinfectant, bleach, or fumigant that will kill the scabies or their eggs. Instead, decontamination occurs by washing all bedding, clothing, and towels in hot water and drying in a hot dryer. Dry cleaning those items is also effective. Further, sealing the items in a plastic bag for at least 72 hours can kill off the scabies; the mites generally do not survive more than two to three days away from human skin.

Additional Considerations

Scabies can occur regardless of a person's hygiene practices or cleanliness. It is not uncommon for scabies to infest large group settings such as college dorms, camps, or nursing homes. Unlike many other STDs, scabies is treatable and be eliminated without lifelong consequences if the treatment regimen is properly followed. Treatment begun as early as possible is key to ensuring that scabies and their eggs are destroyed and minimizes, then, the opportunity to transmit scabies to someone else. Most people with the itching rash of scabies attribute it to some cause other than scabies and try various over-the-counter medications or topical creams and lotions inappropriately. There need not be a stigma surrounding scabies; scabies is part of the natural environment but are traditionally controlled through standard laundering or bathing practices. However, there is no guarantee that with regular bathing and laundering of clothing or bedding that scabies will never occur; one mite is sufficient to begin a cascade that eventually leads to infestation. Successful treatment, then, is available if one seeks evaluations by a health-care practitioner early.

Prevention

Scabies is prevented by avoiding direct skin-to-skin contact with a person infested with scabies, or with their items of clothing or bedding. Treating all persons of the same household, particularly for those who have prolonged skin-to-skin or sexual contact with the person infested, regardless if symptoms are present, is recommended to suppress a potential outbreak. All household members, sexual partners, or contacts, should be treated at the same time to prevent possible reexposure and reinfestation. Bedding and clothing worn or used next to the skin from a person infested at any time during the three days before treatment began should be machine washed and dried using hot water and hot dryer cycles or be dry cleaned. Items that cannot be washed or dry cleaned can be disinfected by storing them in a plastic bag for several days to a week.

Signs, Symptoms, and Diagnosis

35. Does everyone always develop symptoms of an STD?

A majority of STDs are elusive, meaning the disease is present in the body but there are no obvious signs that they are infected with an STD. Therefore, most people will not develop any signs or symptoms of an STD even if they are infected with specific microorganisms that cause STDs. There are a few STDs that have classic symptoms, for example, the foul-smelling discharge associated with trichomoniasis or the intense itching in the genital area associated with "crabs." However, most of the STDs that are caused by bacteria or viruses often go unnoticed and, therefore, undetected.

Bacteria and viruses enter the body through breaks in the skin or direct contact with mucous membranes. The microorganisms, then, can embed themselves in specific body structures such as the cervix of the uterus or the inner lining of the penis. Viruses, further, can enter the bloodstream and remain dormant until certain situations like illness or stress cause biochemical changes in the body that lets the virus "wake up" and become active. Other times bacteria will grow slowly and not cause changes in the body structures they are embedded in until they sufficiently multiply. Regardless, the important commonality that both bacteria and viruses share is that they are living microorganisms that can easily be transmitted, or passed, from person to person even if no symptoms are present.

Unprotected oral, vaginal, or anal sex is the primary way most micro-organisms are transmitted from person to person. However, some viruses like herpes or human papillomavirus (HPV) can be transmitted by skin-to-skin contact. It is easy, then, for microorganisms to reside in a host. Microorganisms, however, can be easily shared; some microorganisms remain with the infected person while some pass on to a new, uninfected person. When this happens, the microorganisms have, essentially, infected two people. Any new partner, further, stands an equal chance of being infected by the same microorganisms.

Screening tests were developed to identify the microorganisms that cause STDs even when no symptoms are present. Specifically, cultures taken from the vagina, cervix, rectum, or the tip and inner lining of the penis can be examined under a microscope to identify specific bacteria, protozoa, or fungus. Additionally, specific laboratory tests can detect the presence of a virus, or a virus' genetic material. Screening tests, then, allow for early treatment to kill off certain microorganisms before both symptoms develop or the microorganism gets passed on to an uninfected person.

36. What are the most common signs and symptoms of an STD?

If a person is infected with an STD, and signs or symptoms are present, he or she is most likely to notice some sort of physical change in his or her body or its normal function. These changes, however, differ between men and women.

Men are most likely to have physical symptoms in the genital area. Specifically, men notice discharge from the tip of the penis that can be clear, white, thick, milky, or yellowish-green. Often the discharge is accompanied by itching at the tip, or immediately within the opening of the penis. The tip of the penis may become reddened or, if uncircumcised, the foreskin may be reddened, irritated, swollen, or difficult to retract. Some men may notice pain only when they urinate with an increased stinging-type pain when the urine stream begins or ends. Additionally, men may also notice lingering discomfort such as burning pain or dull aching along the inside shaft of the penis after urination or following sexual activity.

Women, in contrast, are more likely to notice symptoms earlier than men. If any symptoms are present, women will notice or report irritation, discomfort, or discharge in the vaginal area or at the urinary opening. Typically, women with redness, swelling, skin or vaginal irritation often feel pain, itching, burning, or generalized soreness in the vaginal area. As the STD progresses or worsens, a woman may notice that it is increasingly painful to sit for prolonged periods of time, walk long distances, ride a bicycle, or wear constrictive clothing like tight underwear or pantyhose. When women have this generalized genital discomfort, they often report an odor in the vaginal area or a feeling of uncleanliness that does not go away with showering, powders, or the use of body wash, soaps, deodorant, or perfume. A discharge, if noticed, typically follows that further irritates the vagina or the external genitalia. The discharge can pool at the vaginal opening, or on underpants, a panty liner, or sanitary napkin. The discharge may have its own unique odor that can be fishy or generally malodorous, such as the discharge common with bacterial vaginosis (BV) or possibly gonorrhea or chlamydia.

What is important to distinguish is that symptoms are not always common when an STD is present; many STDs have no symptoms at all and a person is often unaware they are infected. Most STDs, therefore, have no overt symptoms and people can continue to pass the microorganisms that cause STDs from person to person unknowingly.

37. Can I be tested for an STD and how?

Most STDs can be diagnosed through routine screening tests. The tests, however, differ based upon whether the STD is bacterial, viral, fungal, or protozoan in nature.

Bacterial STDs are common and their symptoms, if any, are the most noticeable. For example, if a person is going to have symptoms of a bacterial STD, they are most likely to exhibit symptoms of discharge, itching, burning, or irritation. These symptoms, then, are what typically motivate someone to seek medical evaluation or treatment. During an evaluation for the presence of bacterial STDs, the person will undergo a complete health history and physical examination by a health-care practitioner and testing that includes cultures taken from either the penis or vagina to detect or identify the presence of chlamydia or gonorrhea. For men, this testing may require a culture taken of any discharge that is present or a swab of tip or inner lining of the penis with a cotton-tipped applicator. For women, a pelvic examination is necessary where a speculum is inserted in the vagina to allow visualization and examination of the cervix. The health-care practitioner can then swab the walls of the vagina and the cervix with a specialized cotton-tipped applicator to obtain a culture.

Viral infections, in contrast, can be diagnosed through specific laboratory blood tests or by swabbing and culturing an active lesion that can be analyzed under a microscope in a laboratory to identify specific viruses. The problem, however, is that people experiencing a viral STD have symptoms that mimic other diseases, so testing for specific viral STDs like herpes, HPV, or HIV is often overlooked or not suspected during an initial evaluation. However, if a person presents to a health-care practitioner for treatment of a painful lesion in the genital area, a health-care practitioner may take a culture of the lesion by gently swabbing the area and sending the swab to a laboratory for microscopic analysis where the presence of herpes, or HPV, may be confirmed. Viral illness caused by Hepatitis B, Hepatitis C, or HIV, however, are often diagnosed after all other sources of acute infection have been eliminated. Testing for Hepatitis B, Hepatitis C, and HIV requires laboratory blood tests that can take several days to be resulted.

Fungal or protozoan infections are treated based on the findings of a physical examination (with a pelvic exam included for women) and the symptoms a person is reporting. While the appearance and possible odor of any discharge, the discomfort reported, and any localized skin irritation is convincing enough for a health-care practitioner to implement antifungal or other antibiotic therapy, a sample of any discharge present that is examined under a microscope in an office or clinic can quickly identify some fungi or protozoans. Confirmation and identification of the presence of the specific fungus or protozoan, however, requires a more detailed microscopic analysis in a laboratory.

38. How soon can I be tested for an STD after having unprotected sex?

If someone suspects that they have been exposed to an STD because of unprotected sex, including when condoms break, immediate testing is not an option. Because the microorganisms which lead to STDs need time to multiply or mature to be detectable by current laboratory methods, often a specific amount of time needs to pass following exposure before any meaningful testing or screening can be performed. It is understood that the anxiety that follows an episode of unprotected sex, regardless of the circumstances, can be extreme. However, testing or screening that is done too early or done inappropriately, yields no useful information and can be harmful. Therefore, general testing and screening guidelines have been established.

When a person has an episode of unprotected sex and fears exposure to any of the STDs, a natural inclination is to desire to be "tested for everything." While there is a possibility to test or screen for a majority of STDs, timing is essential. Screening or diagnostic tests that are performed too early may yield a false negative or a false positive result, meaning the results of specific tests can be inaccurate and therefore lead to inadequate, or incorrect, treatment decisions. The microorganisms that cause STDs are not detectable immediately after exposure with current screening or testing mechanisms; the microorganisms, in turn, need time to multiply in order for contemporary testing or screening modalities to detect their presence. Health-care practitioners, then, will often delay screening a person for STDs until a specified period of time has elapsed so the results of any screening or testing can be more accurate to appropriately guide treatment decisions. Screening or testing time frames, then, are different for each of the various microorganisms that cause STDs.

The first, and earliest, STDs a person can be screened for is chlamydia and gonorrhea, usually within two weeks post exposure. Two weeks is typically enough time for sufficient amounts of the bacteria that causes gonorrhea and chlamydia to grow and be properly detectable by current screening methods. Symptoms do not need to be present for proper screening to occur. Similarly, most health-care practitioners will not wait for the results of screening tests to initiate treatment if there is a suspicion that gonorrhea or chlamydia may be present; oral antibiotic treatment will be prescribed that will quickly eradicate gonorrhea, chlamydia, or both. The screening tests, when resulted, will either confirm the diagnosis and justify the treatment prescribed, or find no evidence of microorganisms that cause either disease. The treatment, even if the screening tests are negative, is typically safe and does not cause harm if gonorrhea or chlamydia was not present.

Testing for syphilis, in contrast, is possible from one week to three months post exposure. The microorganism that causes syphilis, *Treponema pallidum* (or *T. pallidum*) requires time to multiply in the bloodstream to be detectable by the first screening laboratory blood test. If the first screening for syphilis is positive, a second, more specific blood test looks directly for the presence of the treponema to confirm the diagnosis. Once the diagnosis is confirmed, treatment with antibiotics immediately follows. Repeat testing to determine the effectiveness of the antibiotic treatment will occur several weeks following the treatment and at subsequent follow-up visits or annual physical examinations with a health-care practitioner.

Viral STDs require time to allow the different viruses time to multiply to be detected by current screening tests. The time frame, however, varies anywhere from six weeks to three months post exposure. Specifically, viral STDs such as HIV or Hepatitis B and C cannot be detected or identified by early screening; false positive and negative results are common when testing is done too early. HIV and both forms of Hepatitis are diagnosed by laboratory blood tests that look specifically for the presence of genetic material unique to each type of virus; early testing will not adequately detect that specific genetic material. In contrast, the herpes virus cannot be detected by conventional laboratory blood tests. Often lesions need to be present so a culture of the fluid or material within or surrounding the lesion can be sent to a laboratory for analysis under a microscope to identify the specific herpes virus and confirm a diagnosis. Treatment, then, depends on the results of the microscopic analysis.

When there is a potential exposure to an STD from unprotected sex, the anxiety associated with the event can be stressful. Since testing guidelines are somewhat rigid, it is understandable, then, why the emphasis has shifted to regular screening of individuals at specified intervals based upon a person's lifestyle or sexual practices. Screening tests performed at regular intervals are more likely to detect STDs sooner than waiting for a window of opportunity for testing to open to secure a diagnosis. Open, honest dialogue, then, with a health-care practitioner will allow a screening plan to be developed based upon each person's unique habits and practices that will facilitate timely diagnosis, and treatment, of STDs should they occur.

39. Is there a test for every STD?

Any STD can be diagnosed through a laboratory test that has been developed to detect specific microorganism that cause each of the individual STDs. Some tests are screening tests meaning the potential to detect the presence of an STD exists but a more confirmatory, specific test is required to make a diagnosis. A diagnostic test, then, accurately confirms the presence of a specific microorganism and, therefore, the STD. The difference, however, is how the screening and confirmatory or diagnostic tests are obtained and whether a bacterial, viral, fungal, or protozoan microorganism is the suspect.

Bacterial microorganisms are diagnosed classically through direct cultures taken from mucous membrane surfaces or from visible discharge from the genital area. A physical examination by a health-care practitioner is required (with a pelvic exam for women) to allow an inspection of the skin surfaces in the genital area to identify the presence of any discharge. During the examination, a soft, cotton-tipped applicator is swabbed across the surfaces of the mucous membranes (e.g., the throat, the opening or the inner 1/3 surface of the penis, the walls of the vagina or opening of the cervix, or the immediate inner lining of the rectum) or through a visible pocket of discharge. The swab is then placed in a medium to promote additional growth of the microorganism that makes identification using a microscope easier and faster.

Fungal and protozoan STDs require testing through a medium similar to bacterial STDs. What differs from bacterial STDs is that fungal and protozoan STDs are typically associated with visible discharge. Swabbing mucous membranes, then, is often unnecessary because a sample of any discharge is sufficient to identify any fungus or protozoan that could be the cause of an STD.

Viral STDs, however, cannot be identified by typical cultures using cotton-tipped swabs that are sent for analysis under a microscope. The physical and pelvic examination by a health-care practitioner is used to collect data about signs or symptoms from multiple body systems. This collection of data, then, helps the health-care practitioner formulate differential diagnoses that may include ruling out the presence of viral STDs like HIV or Hepatitis B or C. Laboratory blood tests, then, are required to diagnose HIV and Hepatitis B or C. Syphilis, though not caused by a virus, is similar to HIV and Hepatitis B or C because a thorough physical examination is required to collect data so an appropriate screening laboratory blood test can occur. If a screening test for syphilis detects the presence of the causative treponema, a more accurate, confirmatory test will identify *Treponema pallidum* (or *T. pallidum*) and treatment, then, will follow. Herpes, in contrast, cannot be diagnosed by laboratory blood tests. There is no way to determine the presence of herpes, further, until symptoms such as lesions in the genital area develop. If genital lesions develop, cultures can be taken directly from the lesions that when analyzed under a microscope will identify herpes simplex virus (i.e., HSV-2) to confirm a diagnosis.

40. Can I tell if someone has an STD before having sex with them?

There is no way to tell if someone has an STD from looking at them. Self-reporting that one is STD-free, further, is unreliable; most people with STDs experience no outward signs or symptoms of a disease, feel well, and falsely assume, then, that they are disease-free. Outward appearances, further, can be deceiving; STDs are not limited to a particular lifestyle, socioeconomic group, gender, or age group.

It is often impossible for an uninfected sex partner to know if a potential, or actual, partner has an STD that can be contagious; symptoms, if any, are often a late sign that an STD is present. It is often these later signs that can possibly serve as a warning to an uninfected partner that an STD may be present. If a person with a bacterial, fungal, or protozoan STD remains untreated, discharge is often present in both men and women (i.e., from the tip of the penis, the vagina, or from the rectum). The discharge can be sticky, often malodorous, and can be copious in amount. The uninfected partner may notice redness or irritation to the infected person's genital skin, or find their potential partner is complaining of frequent itching, burning, or scratching in the genital area. A partner with herpes may complain of increased genital soreness, or avoid touching or foreplay that involves direct contact with the skin surfaces of the genitalia. Viral STDs other than herpes, in contrast, are usually associated with more generalized bodily symptoms such as fever, fatigue, weight loss, or frequent infections. These late signs, again, are rare and often difficult to recognize; as a general rule, there are typically no observable signs, signals, or symptoms, then, which would alert someone that a potential partner has an STD.

A person does not need to have obvious signs or symptoms to transmit an STD to an uninfected partner. Many STDs are spread person-to-person when no symptoms are present. Since there are no obvious signs that a person has an STD, and the fact that anyone can be infected with the microorganisms that cause STDs, there are steps one can take prior to initiating sexual activity to lower one's risk of contracting an STD. First, ask potential partners about their sexual history: Who have they had sex with in the past? Was any of their sexual encounters unprotected oral, vaginal, or anal sex? Have they ever, or at any time, suspected that they might have been exposed to an STD? Have they ever had symptoms of an STD but were never treated? Or has he or she ever been treated for an actual or suspected STD? Importantly, when was their last screening for HIV and what were the results?

Second, condom use is recommended regardless of how a potential partner answers your questions. Irrespective of the length, quality, or intensity of the relationship, potential partners may or may not be forthcoming about the true details of their sexual health history or sexual activities. If a potential partner is honest about his or her sexual health history, one can employ protective measures like condom use and the couple, together, can develop a plan for regular STD screening. If a potential partner is not forthcoming about his or her sexual health history, or if one suspects that a potential partner is not being honest or is leaving out significant health details, condom use, then, affords one protection against a majority of STDs and should, therefore, be used properly and consistently.

Treatment and Prevention

41. What should I do if I think I have an STD?

If a person suspects that he or she was exposed to an STD, or if the person suspects that he or she has symptoms of an STD, an evaluation by a health-care practitioner is essential. An incredible amount of anxiety or embarrassment can surround the realization that an STD is possible and a potential evaluation by a health-care practitioner. However, these feelings are often unnecessary. Health-care practitioners are experienced in managing all aspects of STDs and are sensitive to the fact that situations or circumstances surrounding the diagnosis and treatment of any STD is riddled with fear, nervousness, and uncertainty. Health-care practitioners, then, treat each person individually, holistically, and with discretion and respect.

What one should not do is believe they can treat an STD themselves. There are no over-the-counter preparations available to treat STDs except for products currently available for purchase in a pharmacy or other retail store to treat vaginal yeast infections (which if used inappropriately can mask symptoms of a worsening STD or other condition). Medication prescribed to someone else should never be used or borrowed. Similarly, old prescriptions, including any unused antibiotic pills or topical medicated creams, should be avoided. Home remedies, including herbal supplements, poultices, soaks, or vaginal inserts are often ineffective, can actually worsen the condition, and should, therefore, be avoided. Douching,

showering, or soaking in water with harsh chemicals, soaps, or other products should also be avoided.

Until an evaluation by a health-care practitioner can occur, one should
abstain from sexual activity, especially if symptoms of genital redness or
irritation, pain, itching, burning, or discharge are present. If sexual activity is going to occur, the consistent and proper use of condoms will not
only minimize transmission of an STD to an uninfected partner but also
minimize the introduction or exposure of the genital areas to new bacteria.

Evaluation by a health-care practitioner, then, is essential to a proper
diagnosis and development of an individualized treatment plan if one suspects they have contracted an STD. The health-care practitioner is an
advocate to not only treating an existing STD but also developing a plan
for routine screening exams and follow-up for overall health maintenance.

42. What can happen if an STD isn't treated?

Many STDs have no symptoms at all. The microorganisms that cause STDs
remain within the genital tract, multiply slowly, or may never evolve into
a fulminant infection with classic symptoms such as discharge, lesions, or
discomfort. Despite having no symptoms develop, a person is still capable of transmitting an STD to an infected partner. Further, these microorganisms are still detectable through routine screening and diagnostic
tests even if no symptoms are present. Routine screening tests, then, help
diagnose STDs without symptoms and allow treatment to occur. STDs
that are not treated, however, can have harmful effects on multiple body
systems depending on the disease and its causative microorganism.

The problem with all STDs is the secondary infections they cause both
locally and systemically. For example, localized herpes lesions can lead to more
extensive infection of the surrounding tissues that can be difficult, as well as
painful, to cure. STDs can spread throughout the female and male genital
tracts and lead to infertility, adhesions, or pelvic inflammatory disease (PID).
HIV, in contrast, can continue to multiply and break down the immune system to the point it becomes ineffective, leaving a person unable to combat any
type of infection. Syphilis, similarly, if left untreated can begin to break down
major body organs like the heart, lungs, kidneys, or brain and lead to death.

The most profound similarity among any untreated STD is its potential
to cause permanent damage to other structures, or systems, within the
body. Additionally, the threat of permanent damage to the reproductive
organs, leading to lifelong infertility, is real and can happen easily if STDs
are left untreated. Properly diagnosing, and treating, STDs is essential to

not only eradicate the disease in its early stages but also to ensure protection of other body systems and fertility.

43. Does my partner have to be treated if I have an STD? Or do I have to get treatment if my partner has an STD but I feel OK?

Any time health-care professionals diagnose an STD, the current and previous sex partners of the infected person are considered an important component in the development of an individualized treatment plan. Most STDs require some sort of treatment for current or previous sex partners, while others require sex partners to participate in ongoing screening or surveillance to monitor for the development of an STD. Whether a sex partner requires actual treatment or disease surveillance depends upon whether the STD is bacterial, viral, fungal, or parasitic in origin.

Bacterial STDs such as chlamydia, gonorrhea, or syphilis require treatment with antibiotics to cure the disease in an infected person. Since the infected person often has no symptoms of a bacterial STD, his or her sex partner, then, may also be infected and has no symptoms also. Further, it is often difficult to determine if the infected person contracted a bacterial STD from his or her current or previous sex partners. Because bacterial STDs are easy to transmit between current partners and future partners, it is strongly suggested that current and previous sex partners of a person infected with a bacterial STD be notified and treated. Treatment for current and previous sex partners is typically the same as what is prescribed for an infected person: a brief course of oral antibiotic therapy, education to prevent transmission or reinfection, and a plan for individualized surveillance and STD screening.

Viral STDs such as herpes, HIV, or Hepatitis B or C, have no defined cure or treatment that can eradicate, or prevent, the disease from developing in a sex partner. Because no treatment is available, sex partners of a person infected with a viral STD are encouraged to participate in regular screening tests to identify the presence of disease, if any, as early as possible. Screening tests, however, are only available for HIV and Hepatitis B or C; the presence of herpes, in contrast, can only be determined by sampling material from active lesions identified under a microscope. Treatment plans for viral STDs are individualized for each person and depend upon which disease is diagnosed.

Fungal STDs, such as yeast, typically require only the infected person to be treated. For women, a vaginal yeast infection can occur regardless of sexual activity. However, it is possible for a male sex partner to transmit yeast from one female sex partner to another without having any signs or symptoms of a yeast infection himself. Treatment, then, is often aimed at eradicating the overgrowth of yeast in the infected woman.

Parasitic STDs, such as crabs, require partners to be treated to minimize the spread of the insects or continued reinfestation among or between partners. Crabs are easy to pass from person to person; successful treatment in one partner, however, does not protect him or her from becoming reinfested with crabs again at any time. The only way to minimize reinfestation, then, is to treat both partners at the same time along with the necessary cleaning and disinfecting of clothing, bedding, and other fabrics in both partners' environments. Other sex partners of either infested person should also be treated to prevent similar outbreaks among multiple groups of people.

Notifying sex partners, however, is not always easy. Often there is a stigma associated with telling a sex partner that he or she has potentially been exposed to an STD and that he or she needs to seek an evaluation and treatment from a health-care professional. Since most STDs have no symptoms, a sex partner may ignore the suggestion to seek an evaluation or wait to see if symptoms develop. In order to lessen the burden of notifying sex partners and having them seek treatment, Expedited Partner Treatment (EPT) was developed that allows health-care practitioners to provide a prescription, or actual medication, to the partners of a person diagnosed with specific STDs such as gonorrhea or chlamydia without first examining the partners. While an individualized examination and treatment plan from a health-care practitioner remains the ideal method from managing sex partners of an infected person, EPT has provided a viable option for not only halting the spread of specific STDs among a community but also preventing multiple opportunities for reinfection for the infected person once treatment is completed. Despite the success of EPT at limiting the transmission or reinfection of specific STDs, it is only available in 38 states in the United States as of December 2016; it is potentially allowable in eight states (Alabama, Delaware, Georgia, Kansas, New Jersey, Oklahoma, South Dakota, Virginia) and Puerto Rico, and prohibited in four (Kentucky, New Hampshire, South Carolina, and West Virginia).

Regardless of whether EPT is available or not, health departments across the United States have adopted, and participated in, mandatory reporting of STDs. Health-care practitioners are required, depending upon the state they are practicing in, to notify specific government health agencies when specific STDs are diagnosed. Each state, then, has its own list of reportable STDs but most include gonorrhea, chlamydia, syphilis,

HIV, chancroid, and Hepatitis B or C. Health departments not only use this information to track the incidence and prevalence of specific diseases but also monitor outbreaks or possible epidemics of diseases within individual counties so adequate resources can be allocated to areas in need. Health departments, further, participate in identifying and notifying previous and current sex partners of infected individuals about their possible exposure to an STD. What is important to emphasize is that each person's identity and confidentiality are maintained by state health departments; there is no "Watch List" nor are names released to sex partners when notifications are made. State health departments, further, rely on the trust they develop with counties and the individuals infected with STDs so they take deliberate steps to not violate a person's confidentiality. The state health departments, along with notifying sex partners, also work with them to provide access to testing or treatment services, counseling, education, and any other follow-up testing or surveillance.

44. Can I treat an STD on my own naturally or with over-the-counter medication?

Most STDs are caused by microorganisms that are bacterial, viral, fungal, or parasitic in nature. Most microorganisms, then, require a specific course of antibiotics that is individualized to a person infected with an STD. The antibiotic treatment, further, requires a prescription from a health-care practitioner that is filled and dispensed by a pharmacist. Over-the-counter medications, then, are not available for a majority of the STDs.

There are, however, over-the-counter remedies that may control specific symptoms of STDs and possibly cure or alleviate the problem. For example, there are over-the-counter remedies for vaginal yeast infections, along with topical creams or liquids to treat the symptoms of oral herpes. Antifungal creams and vaginal inserts are available for purchase in most pharmacies or other retail stores where medications are sold. Antifungal preparations have specific instructions for use, often with an emphasis that a woman should seek an evaluation by a health-care practitioner if her symptoms persist or worsen. Similarly, there are over-the-counter shampoos, lotions, or creams that are effective at eliminating crabs. Like the antifungals, preparations to kill lice, and crabs specifically, are only effective if they are used properly according to the manufacturer's instructions and that attention is paid to caring for clothing and bedding in the immediate environment.

While the antifungal and lice-killing preparations may be successful at eliminating specific conditions, over-the-counter medications for oral herpes, in contrast, are only intended to provide relief of pain, swelling, or cracking of herpes lesions that erupt on the lips or along the lip margins. Although these products are advertised to speed healing of the lesion, they are powerless to neither eliminate the lesion nor prevent future lesions from erupting. Further, the use of these preparations does not prevent passing the herpes virus to another uninfected person. Additionally, these products are only for use around the mouth; they are not intended for use within or around the genitals for genital herpes lesions.

Research has begun to explore the effectiveness of herbal products or compounds to relieve the symptoms of STDs or possibly cure them without the use of prescription antibiotics. Data, to date, is weak and suggests that there might be a role for herbal preparations in treating STDs. Examples of natural or herbal remedies and their proposed uses include:

Table 1 Herbal or Natural Compounds Proposed for STDs

Herbal or Natural Compound	Indication for Use/Notes for Use
Garlic	Antiviral; germ-killing properties
Oregano	Oregano oil applied to the skin for herpes outbreaks to speed healing and decrease pain
Echinacea	Boosts immune system; hormonal stimulant to enhance body functions to speed healing
Yogurt	Balance natural pH when ingested regularly; natural probiotic to increase the number of "good" bacteria within the vagina or GI tract to fight diseases
Lemon Juice	Astringent applied to skin to decrease pain, burning, or itching associated with STDs; combined with garlic and ingested orally to fight bacterial or fungal STDs
Goldenseal	Strengthens immune system, aids in detoxifying the body, anti-inflammatory
Neem Tree	Works to decrease pain or discomfort of STDs when steeped in hot water and consumed or added to warm bath water for soaking
Milk Thistle	Contains silymarin, which is proposed to alleviate trichomoniasis and increase overall immunity
Cat's Claw	Contains antibacterial and antifungal properties; cannot be used during pregnancy

It is important to emphasize that the data on herbal or natural remedies is inconclusive and should, therefore, be used cautiously. Research
and data on the effectiveness of prescription antibiotics for treating STDs
remains strong to date; prescription antibiotic therapy, then, remains the
safest and most reliable treatment for most STDs.

45. Are STDs preventable?

Despite the increasing incidence of STDs worldwide, there are ways to
prevent becoming infected with one or passing one onto an uninfected
person. One of the most effective ways of preventing STDs is the proper
and consistent use of condoms with each episode of sexual activity. Condoms, available for both men and women, are the only current form of
barrier protection that protects both partners simultaneously. Further,
condoms are inexpensive, available for sale in various types of stores or
vending machines, and disposable. However, for condoms to be effective,
their proper and consistent use cannot be overemphasized.

Both male and female condoms are individually wrapped to preserve
their integrity and elasticity. A condom with a broken wrapper or one
that has been exposed to air or unrolled should not be used but discarded.
For men, a condom should be applied to an erect penis. The reservoir at
the tip of the condom should be visible; there should be enough room at
the tip of the penis to allow the condom reservoir to collect any ejaculated semen. The condom should be unrolled down the shaft or length
of the penis and end at the base of the penis where the testicles or pubic
hair meet the shaft of the penis. An appropriate-size condom is one that
remains snugly adhered to an erect penis and does not roll around or off
the penis freely. The fit should be comfortable and not painfully tight
or constrictive on any part of the penis. Before use, a condom can be
lubricated with a water-based lubricant or spermicide cream or jelly; other
products like baby oil, cooking oils or vegetable shortenings, petroleum
jelly, saliva, or oil-based lubricant should be avoided because they can
potentially break down the integrity of a condom and cause the condom
to break. Further, use of products other than water-based lubricants to
lubricate a condom has no spermicidal effect and can cause injury or
discomfort to a sex partner during sexual activity. Once vigorous sexual
activity has begun, it is important to check that the condom is still properly applied and not rolling up or loosening. If no ejaculation occurs, and
the condom is still intact, additional lubricant can be applied and the
condom used for an additional episode of sexual activity. If the condom

is removed, it should never be reapplied. If ejaculation does occur, care should be taken when the penis is withdrawn from the vagina or rectum; the base of the condom should be held firmly prior to withdrawing to avoid leaking any seminal fluid then removed and discarded.

Female condoms, in contrast, require a different approach for use because they are inserted into the vagina prior to use. Like male condoms, female condoms are available in a range of sizes. The inner ring at the closed end of the sheath is used to insert the condom inside the vagina and hold it in place during sex. The rolled outer ring at the open end of the sheath remains outside the vagina and covers part of the external genitalia. To use the female condom, a small amount of water-based lubricant is applied on the outside of the closed end of the sheath. A woman can either lie down, squat, or stand with one foot up on a chair or the toilet to position herself properly to insert the condom. The inner ring at the closed end is squeezed and inserted into the vagina similar to the way a woman would insert a tampon. The inner ring is pushed gently into the vagina as far as it can go, typically until it reaches the cervix. As the fingers are removed from the vagina, the sheath unrolls and the outer ring hangs about an inch outside the vagina. During sexual activity or intercourse, it is normal for the female condom to move side to side; intercourse should be stopped if the penis slips between the condom and the walls of the vagina. If ejaculation has not occurred, a female condom can be gently removed from the vagina to add additional spermicide or lubricant then reinserted into the vagina. If ejaculation occurs, the outer ring can be squeezed and twisted to contain any semen within the pouch then gently removed from the vagina and discarded. Female condoms should not be rinsed, rerolled or stored for future use.

While condoms provide the most effective barrier method to prevent STDs, abstinence from all oral, vaginal, or anal sexual activity or intercourse remains the only proven method to avoid getting or giving an STD. While complete abstinence is not always feasible, safer sex practices like mutual masturbation or other forms of physical intimacy without oral, vaginal, or anal penetration or an exchange of potentially infectious bodily fluids can be satisfying to both partners. Regardless of whether condoms or other forms of prevention are used, regular screening for STDs still needs to occur to allow prompt treatment of any STD and prevent transmission to an uninfected partner.

46. Does douching after sex minimize my chances of getting an STD?

Women use douches to clean the vagina and eliminate odors or debris. Typically, women opt to douche at the end of a menstrual period or as a part of hygiene practices that are dictated by cultural or religious traditions or rituals. Douching, however, can be harmful and current scientific evidence supports that it does not prevent pregnancy or STDs.

Because the act of douching requires a forceful stream of water or chemicals to be squeezed into the vagina, sperm or microorganism that cause STDs that are in the vagina can, therefore, be pushed by the stream of liquid from the douche past the cervix and into the uterus itself. Additionally, the soaps, fragrances, or other chemicals in the douching liquid can irritate the vaginal walls or cervix and create multiple portals of entry for STD-causing microorganisms. Further, douching can kill off the natural, healthy microorganism (or flora) that live in the vagina and, therefore, expose a woman to other vaginal infections. Douching, then, cannot prevent an STD from occurring and can actually be harmful to a woman if performed regularly.

It is important to emphasize for both men and women that attempting to clean, swab, soak, or scrub the vagina, penis, or anus with soaps, detergents chemicals or hot liquids will also not prevent STDs from occurring and can, similar to douching, pose significant harm to both men and women. There are no over-the-counter products or chemicals available that are intended to be used to clean, rinse, or lavage any body cavity or opening to prevent STDs from occurring. Further, all products like detergents, soaps, cleaners, or antiseptic solutions are clearly labeled "For External Use Only" and therefore not meant to be ingested orally or inserted in any way into the mouth, penis, vagina, or rectum. Further, use of any harsh product in a manner other than what it is intended for can cause severe burns, ulcerations, infections, or permanent damage to skin or mucous membranes. While regular bathing or showering is recommended for overall health and maintenance of good hygiene, douching is not supported by current research and therefore is not recommended for use to prevent any STD.

47. Do lubricants or spermicides decrease my chances of contracting an STD?

Lubricants and spermicidal cream or jelly are intended for use during sexual activity. Lubricants add extra moisture to sexual activity or intercourse to make the vagina or rectum more smooth or slippery to allow ease and comfort of penetration. Spermicides, in contrast, are intended to kill sperm cells so they do not enter the cervix and cause pregnancy. Spermicides may be added into a lubricant by a manufacturer and, therefore, serve a dual purpose during sex to both prevent pregnancy and enhance sexual activity or intercourse. Lubricants, in contrast, are not always spermicidal.

Lubricants and spermicidal cream or jelly have a role in STD prevention because they minimize the amount of friction that occurs during sexual activity or intercourse. While friction during sexual activity heightens arousal and eventually helps both partners achieve orgasm, friction also causes skin and mucous membrane tissues to dry out, crack, tear, or split. These breaks, regardless of their size, in the integrity of the skin surfaces or mucous membranes are potential portals of entry for harmful microorganisms, including those that cause STDs. Lubricants and spermicide cream or jelly, then, keep skin and mucous membrane surfaces greasy or slippery so friction is greatly reduced, thereby minimizing breaks in the skin or mucous membranes' integrity.

Lubricants and spermicides do not contain any antibiotics; they do not kill any of the microorganisms that cause STDs. Spermicides, in turn, only destroys sperm cells that can cause a pregnancy to occur. While lubricants and spermicides are intended to enhance sexual activity, some of the current formulations of both that are available for purchase can cause various skin or mucous membrane reactions that can lead to rashes, swelling, or discomfort. Since these reactions can further lead to breakdown of the skin or the integrity of the mucous membrane surfaces, it is suggested that small dabs of lubricant or spermicide be tested on various skin surfaces prior to using for sexual activity or intercourse. Further, for people with known sensitivity or reactions in general, it is advised to avoid using the variety of lubricants or spermicides that are flavored, scented, warming, or color-enhanced that is currently available for purchase.

48. Is there anything I can do through diet, exercise, or taking supplements to minimize my chances of getting an STD?

There is no specific diet or nutrition plan that will minimize one's chances of contracting an STD. Similarly, neither exercise nor the use of dietary supplements prevents one from getting, or giving an uninfected partner, an STD. However, current research supports that the combination of a nutritious diet and regular exercise supports a healthy immune system that help boost the body's natural infection-fighting abilities. What is important to emphasize, despite the current support for good health through nutrition and exercise, is that a healthy individual is still susceptible to contracting an STD and suffer the same side effects or consequences from an untreated STD. Good nutrition and exercise, then, are thought to support the balance of natural healthy flora within the body and the resilience of body tissues to remain intact as a first line of defense or protection against the harmful microorganisms that cause STDs.

What constitutes good nutrition or the proper amount of exercise varies for each person. However, it is generally accepted that, across different races and cultures, diets that are rich in key nutrients contribute to overall good health. The current trend of "Clean Eating" encompasses a lifestyle that ensures people get the right amount of naturally occurring nutrients (i.e., vitamins and minerals) and avoid current products that deplete the body of nutrients. When the body loses nutrients, or takes few in, the susceptibility to illness is increased.

Vitamins and minerals are easy to consume because they are abundant in the United States through food sources. In a diet that is low in saturated fats and rich in whole grains, fruits, vegetables, and protein, sufficient amounts of vitamins (especially vitamins A, B, C, D, and E) and minerals (specifically selenium, zinc, and iron) are readily available and often existing in their natural form. Diets that contain adequate quantities from each food group, then, are encouraged for maintenance of a healthy immune system.

There are, however, several food types or sources that are believed to not only be lacking in nutritional value or content but also deplete the body of any nutrient stores it may already have. Processed foods, while convenient and affordable, are high in chemical additives, fats, salt, and refined sugars. These foods typically contain artificial flavors, sweeteners, or colors and tend to be fatty or fried. Similarly, refined foods, which cause fluctuations in hormone levels and metabolism of nutrients in the body, are found in a variety of common foods in the form of white flour, sugars, high fructose corn syrup or trans fats. Currently, GMOs, or genetically modified organisms, are plants or animals that have been genetically engineered by adding DNA, hormones, antibiotics, steroids or other chemicals from sources such as bacteria, viruses, or other plants and animals. The organisms that result are often things that would not normally have occurred in nature or through traditional crossbreeding. GMOs, even when digested, are thought to leave material behind in the body that is never excreted nor destroyed, which can lead to organ damage or immune system disorders. A diet, then, that is a combination of processed and refined foods, along with GMOs, is thought to destroy the immune system by weakening the body's natural protective barriers and its ability to fight off infections. Further, the ability of the body to utilize prescription antibiotics if prescribed to treat an existing infection or other condition is greatly diminished. The solution, then, although not always feasible, is to select organically certified foods that are GMO-free, not processed, and without refined products.

The intake of alcohol and the use of illegal drugs also play a key role in minimizing the body's ability to prevent infections. Alcohol use drains the body of key nutrients as more vitamins and minerals are needed by the body to help metabolize any alcohol ingested. With repeated alcohol use or episodes of binge drinking there is a higher likelihood of vomiting, decreased appetite, and poor food intake. Similarly, food choices made while drinking alcohol are often processed foods or those containing refined products. Specific to STDs, the use of alcohol can lower one's inhibitions and critical thinking, thereby contributing to sexual activity or intercourse on an impulse or without the use of condoms. Illegal drug use, like alcohol, also tends to suppress the appetite and often requires a significant amount of calories and stored nutrients to metabolize the drug. Similar to alcohol use, being under the influence of drugs can contribute to unintended, promiscuous, or risky sexual activity or intercourse. Further, the use of intravenous (IV) drugs exposes a person to the risk of contracting blood-borne diseases like HIV and Hepatitis B or C.

49. Can STDs be transmitted through oral sex?

The microorganisms that cause STDs rely on tissues like mucous membranes to grow and flourish. Mucous membranes, then, make up the outside skin and moist internal lining of the penis, vagina, and anus. These same mucous membranes, further, are found on the lips and inside the mouth and throat. Oral sex is defined as anytime the lips, mouth, or tongue comes in contact with a man's penis (i.e., fellatio), a woman's genitals including the clitoris, vaginal opening, or the skin surrounding the vagina (i.e., cunnilingus), or the anus of another person (i.e., anilingus or "rimming"). Having oral sex, then, can make the skin, or mucous membranes, in both the oral and genital areas vulnerable to irritation, abrasions, or small tears that can allow the microorganisms that cause STDs to be passed between partners.

Many STDs, as well as other infections, can be spread through oral sex. Anyone exposed to an infected partner can contract an STD in the mouth, throat, genitals, or rectum. The risk of getting, or spreading, an STD through oral sex, then, depends on several factors including the specific STD, the sex act practiced and how often it is performed, and how common or prevalent a specific STD is among the population. The most common

STDs that are passed through oral sex, then, include, but not limited to, human papillomavirus (HPV), herpes, chlamydia, gonorrhea, and HIV.

HPV has become increasingly more common in the United States. There are over 40 strains of HPV that live solely on the mucous membranes, with several strains leading to an increased risk of cancers many years after exposure. HPV, then, can be passed easily from person to person during oral sex. HPV thrives in the moist mucous membranes of the mouth and throat. While there are no obvious symptoms of an oral HPV infection, the virus can live for years within the mouth or throat and predispose a person to developing cancers of the tongue or throat in the future.

Herpes, including HSV-1 (which most commonly causes cold sores in or around the mouth) and HSV-2 (which most commonly causes genital herpes) can live and flourish well in both the mouth and the genital areas. Further, oral sex can transfer viruses to or from the mouth and the genital areas. While herpes is most likely to be passed from person to person when there are blisters or sores present, it can be easily passed when there are no obvious lesions also. Performing oral sex on a partner with genital herpes, then, can pass either type of HSV to a partner and lead to oral herpes. Similarly, receiving oral sex from a partner with oral herpes can spread either type of HSV and cause genital herpes.

Chlamydia and gonorrhea, the most common bacterial STDs, are both highly contagious and, therefore, easily passed between partners through oral sex and lead to infections of the mouth or throat. The risk of contracting chlamydia, gonorrhea, or both, is higher with fellatio compared to cunnilingus, especially when there is ejaculation, then oral contact or swallowing, of infected semen. Gonorrhea in the throat, typically, does not cause any symptoms but sometimes causes a sore throat or painful swallowing like strep throat. Chlamydia in the throat, conversely, rarely causes any signs or symptoms and, like gonorrhea, will continue to grow and flourish unnoticed.

HIV, although not typically a virus that lives on the mucous membranes, thrives in the blood, semen, vaginal secretions, or other body fluids. Contact with these bodily fluids during oral sex, then, is what puts a person at risk for contracting HIV. Specifically, cuts, tears, sores or unhealthy gums in the mouth can be portals of entry for the HIV virus for the person giving oral sex. Similarly, for the person receiving oral sex, any areas of broken skin in or around the genitals serve as potential portals of entry for the HIV virus if there is contact with blood or secretions from the mouth.

Oral sex can be a mutually safe, satisfying sexual experience if both partners take precautions to protect each other from transmitting STDs. While abstinence from oral, vaginal, or anal sex remains the only way to prevent transmission of STDs between partners, the proper and consistent use of both male or female condoms, including for oral sex, is currently the most effective barrier method to prevent the spread of STDs. Additionally, oral sex with a partner who is mutually monogamous and has participated in regular STD screening or testing and remains uninfected further minimizes the risk of transmitting or contracting STDs. Avoiding oral contact with body fluids, especially blood in or around the mouth, vagina, or anus, seminal fluid ("pre-cum") or ejaculated semen (including the swallowing of ejaculated semen) can also decrease one's risk of contracting an STD from a partner.

50. If I have an STD, am I contagious?

Whether or not an STD is contagious depends upon the individual STD and the microorganism that causes it. Often people define the word "contagious" to mean that a sick person is able to cause a healthy person to contract an illness, or the symptoms of an illness, from being in close proximity with them or by sharing living space. Additionally, people can often contract an illness if they are contaminated by a sick individual from sharing utensils, touching surfaces a sick person touched, or being touched by a sick person through a hug, kiss, or a handshake. While these types of contact can, indeed, spread the viruses or bacteria that cause such things as the common cold, strep throat, or the flu, STDs are not passed from person to person by social or public contact. STDs, in contrast, are often passed through intimate sexual contact where there is an opportunity for the microorganisms that cause STDs to come in contact with broken skin or susceptible mucous membranes, thereby leading to specific infections. The various STDs, then, are contagious in different ways and within different time periods.

Gonorrhea and chlamydia are the most highly contagious during times of intimate sexual activity. Because most people are unaware that they are infected with gonorrhea, chlamydia, or both, they often forget to use barrier methods such as condoms and, therefore, pass the microorganism *N. gonorrhea*, *C. trachomatis*, or both, to an uninfected partner during oral, vaginal, or anal sexual intercourse. Even simple sexual contact, for example, genital skin-to-skin contact where the tip of the penis touches the outside of the vagina or rectum, can often be enough to transmit microorganisms that cause STDs to, or between, uninfected partners. Symptoms of gonorrhea or chlamydia, then, can become apparent any-where from two days to one month post exposure. What is important to remember with any STD, including gonorrhea and chlamydia, is that physical signs or symptoms do not need to be present to transmit the dis-ease to an uninfected partner; most STDs, in fact, are transmitted when no symptoms are present at all.

Some STDs do not require oral, vaginal, or anal intercourse to be transmitted. Skin-to-skin contact, without oral, vaginal, or anal pene-tration, can often be sufficient to transmit specific STDs from an infected person to an uninfected partner. For example, herpes, crabs, or mollus-cum contagiosum are easily spread from person to person when the skin or skin lesions of the infected person rubs against, or comes in contact with breaks or tears regardless of size, in the skin of an uninfected person. Viruses or insects, then, transmit easily from person to person and do not require intercourse or breaks in the mucous membrane tissues for an infec-tion to occur. Similar to gonorrhea and chlamydia, viral or insect-borne infections such as herpes, crabs or molluscum contagiosum often have no symptoms during the first several days, or weeks, following the onset of infection so unknowingly transmitting a specific disease, then, is easy. Symptoms of viral or insect-borne STDs, further, can take anywhere from one to two weeks to develop post exposure or transmission.

Other STDs, such as HIV or syphilis, require contact with infected body fluids, such as semen, vaginal secretions, or blood, directly with breaks in mucous membranes or skin surfaces to spread the virus or bac-teria that cause each specific disease. Unlike most other STDs, HIV or syphilis requires unprotected oral, vaginal, or anal sex to transmit their causative microorganisms to an uninfected person. Casual contact, or skin-to-skin sexual contact, then, is not likely to transmit the viruses or bacteria that cause either disease. The duration of sexual contact, however, is irrelevant; HIV or syphilis can be transmitted to an unin-fected person following a brief, singular unprotected sexual encounter. Symptoms of HIV or syphilis, further, can take several weeks to develop. Whereas symptoms of syphilis, such as a chancre, may appear anywhere from 21 to 90 days post exposure, the initial symptoms of HIV may take several months to develop and then several weeks after to be diagnosed. The need for practicing safer sex, along with routine screening for STDs, cannot be overemphasized.

Fortunately, the spread or transmission of most STDs can be greatly minimized by the proper and consistent use of barrier methods such as the male or female condom. Condoms primarily prevent any infected body fluid (e.g., semen or vaginal secretions) from coming in contact with susceptible mucous membrane tissues of the mouth, penis, vagina, or rectum. Condoms alone, however, are insufficient to singularly control the spread of the microorganisms that cause STDs. Regular follow-up with a health-care practitioner that includes frequent STD screenings for all sexually active people, coupled with early treatment for any suspected STDs, and regular use of condoms diminishes the likelihood of transmitting any STDs from one partner to another.

51. Do uncircumcised men transmit STDs more?

There is an ongoing debate within the medical, nursing, and public health communities about the role uncircumcised men play in the spread, or transmission, of STDs. While some health-care experts believe the presence of the male foreskin has no impact on the amount of microorganisms a man may carry in or around the tip of the penis, a fair amount of health-care experts, conversely, maintain the opinion that the foreskin creates an optimum environment to promote the growth, and over-growth, of harmful microorganisms, including those that cause STDs. The data used to support each side of this ongoing argument is based upon the incidence rates of STDs in specific geographic regions. In areas where rates of STD infection are high, circumcision for males is often not performed as a cultural norm or religious ritual. Where rates of STD infection are lowest, a higher proportion of the male population are circumcised compared to other areas of the world. What weakens the argument overall is that STDs continue to occur in both circumcised and uncircumcised men, and in both their male or female partners.

Every male baby is born with a foreskin. The purpose of the foreskin is to protect and cover the head of the penis, or the glans penis. The foreskin is a double-layered fold of skin comprised of smooth muscle tissue, blood vessels, mucous membranes, and sensory neurons. The foreskin is moveable and retracts over the head of the penis, especially when the penis is erect or during sexual intercourse. The foreskin provides lubrication, then, to the tip of the penis and, therefore, helps permit easier entry of the penis into the vagina or rectum. It is proposed that the presence of the foreskin, especially when its retracted back over with an erect penis, heightens sexual pleasure or sensation for both men and women.

Many cultures, however, choose to remove the foreskin from infant males and boys or young men. Residual urine, sweat, and natural lubricant the foreskin produces can accumulate and develop into an adherent, malodorous white substance called smegma. While most uncircumcised men can easily retract their foreskin, especially during bathing or showering, some men are unable to retract the foreskin because it hardens over time and becomes a thick, constrictive, painful band of skin. Because of the potential hygiene and health issues, religious significance, or the growing social disdain for the appearance of an uncircumcised penis by both men and women alike, circumcision remains a frequent surgical procedure worldwide.

The existing body of scientific literature, however, demonstrates that the risk of contracting an STD is less likely with circumcised men. Researchers continue to support the notion that the foreskin can harbor infectious microorganisms that cause STDs and the warm, moist environment provided by the foreskin, coupled with the natural secretions the foreskin provides, helps support and nourish those harmful microorganisms and, therefore, allows them to flourish.

Normal hygiene practices reduce the amount of secretions and surface bacteria that may be growing or hidden under the foreskin. When a man bathes or showers, he should gently retract the foreskin and clean the tip of the penis and surrounding skin with soap and water. While normal bathing will not wash away any of the microorganisms that cause STDs, it can make the environment at the tip of the penis less conducive to the increased growth of microorganisms. The regular and consistent use of condoms, then, is the only effective way for both circumcised and uncircumcised men to prevent transmitting any harmful microorganisms that may be present at or within the tip of the penis, or becoming exposed to harmful microorganisms himself from an infected partner.

Circumcision is a personal choice that is heavily laden in culture, religion, or ritual. All men, however, are capable of transmitting or being exposed to harmful microorganisms regardless of whether a foreskin is present or not. Regular hygiene practices, while recommended for all men, do not minimize a man's risk of transmitting, or being exposed to, harmful microorganisms that cause STDs. Both men and women, then, should insist upon, and practice, the regular and consistent use of condoms to provide the best protection against transmitting, or contracting, STDs.

❖

Case Studies

CASE 1: CHRISTINE

Christine is a 22-year-old woman who recently graduated with honors from college. During her last year of college, she was busy trying to complete all her necessary course requirements to graduate, finish a senior year internship that was directly related to her major, work part time as a waitress in a local restaurant, and maintain a relationship with a new boyfriend. Fortunately, Christine was able to handle her hectic schedule throughout her time in college and deliberately ate well, got exercise and rest, and stayed healthy. Her college offered an on-site student health service that Christine took advantage of on the few rare occasions she became sick. Upon graduation, however, Christine's ability to access the student health service would end as she would be entering the job market, obtaining health insurance of her own, and establishing herself with a health-care practitioner to provide her primary and gynecologist (GYN) care.

Christine's work during her senior year internship allowed her to get hired by a prestigious financial company within a major city. Excited at the prospect of her new job, Christine moved to a new city and into her own apartment but needed to break off her relationship with her college boyfriend. After starting her new job, Christine began exploring her new surroundings, made new friends, and developed a new social network of people her own age. Christine and her friends came to enjoy the nightlife of the city, which included going to new restaurants or bars, listening to live music, or going to dance clubs. Christine was also meeting different men and went out on several dates. While Christine met men she liked, she was focused on her career and opted not to get into a serious relationship with anyone. However, she had sex twice with one man she had dated since arriving in the new city.

After Christine had been working for several months, she realized she had not had an annual physical examination since early in her junior year of college. Through her health insurance, she was able to find a GYN and scheduled an appointment for a complete physical examination. Christine also wanted to explore starting on birth control to protect her against pregnancy, while she continued to date men socially and, occasionally, have sex.

Christine met with her new GYN physician. The physician took time to get to know Christine by asking her a series of questions about her health or illnesses in the past as part of a comprehensive health history. The physician asked Christine, then, about any past illnesses or operations she had, medications she used in the past, and if she had any current allergies to medicines or food. The physician inquired about the health of Christine's family members and probed with questions about any familial diseases like cancers or genetic disorders. The physician asked many questions about Christine's diet, exercise habits, alcohol intake, sleep habits, smoking or tobacco use, and her general safety practices such as seatbelt use, cell phone use while driving, or use of a helmet while bicycling. Lastly, the physician asked Christine specific questions about her sexual health, including the number of partners she has had, number of episodes of unprotected sex, menstrual history, birth control plans, and her fertility plans for the future.

Because Christine was forthcoming with her physician about the number of different sex partners she had since her last GYN exam, her lack of any symptoms of an STD, and that sometimes she has unprotected sex, the physician performed a thorough pelvic examination as part of her physical examination of Christine. The physician found nothing abnormal as she visualized the vagina or cervix or when she palpated Christine's uterus, fallopian tubes, or ovaries. Regardless of her lack of findings, the physician obtained a Pap smear from the cervix and also cultures for gonorrhea and chlamydia using a laboratory swab that gently took cells from inside the cervix with a soft-tipped applicator. After the exam, Christine made a follow-up appointment to speak with the physician about her test results and to discuss her birth control options.

At the follow-up appointment, Christine was surprised to learn she had tested positive for chlamydia. The physician reassured Christine that many sexually active women test positive for chlamydia, gonorrhea, or both, and that the majority of both men and women with chlamydia have no symptoms of the disease. The physician further reassured Christine that the disease was treatable and prescribed a one-time dose of the anti-biotic azithromycin. The physician discussed the need for Christine to notify her previous sex partners so they, too, could be treated and not pass on the disease to other partners. The physician offered to help Christine notify her previous partners or refer them to clinics or other health-care practitioners for proper evaluation and STD screening. Lastly, the physi-cian provided Christine a sample of condoms and told her to use them for all future sexual activity, even if she opts to use additional form of birth control, in order to fully protect herself from future STDs.

Analysis

Christine, like many women, had no signs or symptoms that would have alerted her that she had chlamydia. Additionally, she believed, incor-rectly, that maintaining a healthy lifestyle would shield her from any sort of diseases, including STDs. Men, similarly, are equally as asymptomatic if they are infected with chlamydia; most likely one episode of unprotected sex, then, was sufficient to expose Christine to the harmful bacteria, C. *trachomatis* and, therefore, develop chlamydia.

All sexually active men and women, then, should have a health-care practitioner that they see regularly to evaluate their overall health and perform STD screenings as needed. Since signs and symptoms of chla-mydia are rare, sensitive laboratory tests such as a cervical swab for women or a culture from the tip of the penis in men are the only reliable methods to confirm the presence of any disease and, therefore, guide pre-scribing appropriate treatment. Chlamydia responds well, and quickly, to oral antibiotics such as a single dose of azithromycin or a week's worth of doxycycline. Treatment, however, does not protect a man or woman from being reinfected again. It is necessary, then, to treat all previous (from six months to possibly one year) and current sex partners to prevent further transmission of chlamydia or other STDs (e.g., gonorrhea) and encourage them to seek regular STD screenings.

The proper and consistent use of condoms is the only effective barrier method to prevent transmitting harmful STD-causing microorganisms from partner to partner, including chlamydia. Condoms, then, should be used for all episodes of sexual activity, regardless if other forms of birth control are being used. Birth control only prevents pregnancy and is, therefore, powerless against the harmful microorganisms that cause STDs so the added protection of condoms is beneficial.

CASE 2: ALEX

Alex is a 17-year-old high school senior. Throughout high school, Alex was popular and had a host of male and female friends. Since Alex was active in school clubs and some sports, his network of friends and new contacts continued to grow. Alex dated girls regularly and began having sex in his sophomore year. At first, his sexual activity consisted of receiving oral sex from girls he dated. Later, he began having sexual intercourse with girls he dated or ones he "hooked up" with at parties. These unplanned encounters often meant neither Alex nor his date had condoms with them so sex often occurred unprotected.

During senior year, however, Alex found himself attracted to his male friends or other boys in his class. While Alex had primarily only dated girls, he could not deny the attraction he felt toward certain males but continued to have the same sexual or physical attraction toward girls that he always had. Despite Alex's high school being open and accepting of diversity among the students, Alex did not immediately take advantage of the opportunity to explore a sexual relationship with another boy.

Alex kept his interest in both boys and girls a secret until he met another schoolmate in his theater club who admitted to Alex that he, too, had similar feelings for other boys in school. Alex confided in his friend that he shared the same feelings and, within a short period of time, Alex and his new friend from the theater club developed a closer, more personal relationship. As their relationship grew, they began to spend more time together and started experimenting with sexual activity. What began as simple kissing or touching progressed to oral sex and eventually mutual anal sex that was frequently unprotected. While Alex was exploring a new relationship with another boy, he continued to date, and be sexually active with, girls. Alex tried to remember to use condoms with each sexual encounter but he was not always successful; several of his sexual encounters with girls, then, were unprotected.

One morning Alex awoke and when he attempted to urinate in the bathroom he had difficulty starting his stream of urine. When he was finally able to urinate, he noticed that his urine burned as it passed through the tip of his penis, and that the act of urinating, overall, was painful. Later, while Alex was in school, he noticed his penis was itchy and he constantly felt wetness at the tip. In the bathroom, Alex pulled back his underwear and noticed a white to yellowish-green discharge at the tip of his penis and similar colored stain on his underwear. The discharge felt slightly sticky when Alex touched it and had a strange, strong odor when he sniffed it.

Alex went to the school's library and used the computer to search the Internet for answers that could explain the symptoms he was experiencing. Immediately, the Internet search took him to various websites and information sources about STDs. Alex was nervous that he might have an STD but knew he needed to be seen by a health-care practitioner to identify what was happening to him. Searching further on the Internet, Alex located a clinic that was in a neighboring community.

At the clinic, Alex met a nurse practitioner who listened carefully to Alex's complaints. The nurse practitioner asked Alex questions about his medical and surgical history, along with specific questions about Alex's sexual history, including the number of partners he currently had, his use of condoms, and the types of sexual activity he engaged in. The nurse practitioner performed a physical examination and took note of the creamy white to yellow discharge at the tip of Alex's penis. The nurse practitioner explained his findings to Alex and explained that a simple culture of the discharge was needed to confirm his diagnosis. The nurse practitioner then gently inserted a thin cotton-tipped swab into the opening of Alex's penis, took a sample of the discharge, and placed the swab in a special transport medium so it could be sent to a lab for analysis. The nurse practitioner diagnosed Alex with gonorrhea and told him he was going to prescribe treatment for both gonorrhea and chlamydia because both diseases, especially with Alex's history of unprotected sex with different partners, could be existing simultaneously. After the nurse practitioner reviewed the different treatment options, including a one-time injection of antibiotics or a prescription of antibiotic pills that could be taken over several days, Alex opted for the one-time injection of antibiotics, which the nurse practitioner administered. The nurse practitioner then educated Alex further on the need to use condoms for all his future sexual encounters with both males and females, the need to participate in regular STD screenings, and recommended Alex notify his sex partners of his gonorrhea diagnosis so they, too, could be screened and seek treatment.

Analysis

Gonorrhea, like most of the STDs, has no noticeable symptoms at the onset. Alex was fortunate to notice the burning urination, penile itching, and discharge so he could seek an evaluation and obtain treatment. Chlamydia, then, is often present along with gonorrhea, and present with no symptoms or ones like gonorrhea. Practitioners, then, will often initiate treatment immediately and not wait for cultures to be analyzed in a lab based upon the presenting signs or symptoms. Chlamydia and gonorrhea, then, can be eradicated by powerful antibiotics, for example, Ceftriaxone, given by a one-time injection or through a course of oral tablets taken over several days. While the one-time injection may be temporarily painful, it guarantees rapid delivery of the medication and avoids the need, and cost, for filling a prescription at a pharmacy.

Alex's unprotected oral, vaginal, and anal sexual activity with both men and women exposed him to multiple harmful microorganisms that cause STDs. In turn, Alex exposed his sexual partners to the same harmful microorganisms. The nurse practitioner was correct, then, in emphasizing the importance and need for Alex to use condoms with each of his sexual encounters. Because Alex was having sex with multiple partners, the need for Alex to participate in regular STD screenings, including for HIV, would help diagnose STDs sooner and allow Alex, and his sex partners, to obtain appropriate treatment sooner.

CASE 3: MICHAEL

Michael is a 21-year-old part-time college student who works full time as a waiter. Michael's hours are erratic and he primarily works the evening shift where he is regularly busy managing the dinner and bar crowds. While Michael eats a healthy diet, consumes minimal alcohol, and exercises, he readily admits balancing his long work hours and school schedule often leave him feeling fatigued and in need of sleep.

Michael has been in a mutually monogamous relationship with his girlfriend for three years. Michael had dated several girls throughout high school, including two that he had sex with regularly. Michael and his girlfriend plan to move in together and eventually marry, once they both finish college.

Michael was working his usual shift at the restaurant on a particularly busy Friday. While Michael could keep up with what his customers wanted, he was feeling increasingly more tired as his shift wore on. When his shift ended, Michael went home and went directly to bed. The next morning Michael still felt run down and worried he might be coming down with a cold. When he went to the bathroom after waking up, however, he suddenly felt a burning sensation inside the opening at the tip of his penis. When the burning subsided, Michael worried he might possibly have a urinary tract or bladder infection so he drank copious amounts of water to flush out his system.

With the increased water intake Michael needed to urinate more often; the burning with urination continued. While at work, Michael began to experience soreness and a stinging sensation at the tip of his penis, especially when his underwear rubbed across, or came in contact with, the tip of his penis. Michael began to become concerned because these were symptoms he never experienced before. When Michael finished work, he went home and used a flashlight to examine his penis. Michael noticed redness and small bumps at the tip of his penis, along with small, linear lesion, like a paper cut. Michael called his girlfriend and told her how he was feeling and what he found when he examined the tip of his penis with the flashlight. His girlfriend became concerned also and suggested Michael see his physician.

Michael was able to get an appointment with his physician the next day. Michael described his symptoms and findings in detail to his physician. The physician then did a thorough physical examination of Michael, carefully assessing each body system to find answers to explain Michael's fatigue and discomforts. The physician used a lighted magnifying lens to better visualize the opening at the tip, and the shaft, of Michael's penis. Discovering the same lesion Michael found, the physician sent a special swab that would identify viruses specifically to the lab.

The physician diagnosed Michael with genital herpes. Based upon Michael's physical symptoms of feeling run down, and painful urination coupled with the lesion he could visualize, the physician felt confident that his diagnosis was correct. The physician prescribed antiviral medication for Michael to alleviate most of Michael's symptoms and lessen the duration of the current outbreak. The physician advised Michael that the antiviral medications were not a cure; Michael would continue to have recurrent outbreaks of genital herpes, especially if his body is under stress or during times of illness. Michael was reassured, however, that he would learn to identify symptoms of impending outbreaks and, therefore, be able to start his antiviral medication sooner. The physician further advised Michael to avoid sexual activity during recurrent outbreaks and to have his girlfriend share Michael's diagnosis of genital herpes with her gynecologist or health-care practitioner so she, too, could be monitored or tested for genital herpes. Lastly, the physician informed Michael that if he began to have more frequent, recurrent outbreaks of genital herpes, suppression therapy with antiviral medications could be trialed.

Analysis

Genital herpes is a painful STD that is characterized by outbreaks of herpes lesions anywhere in the genital area. Genital herpes lesions are easily irritated by urine, menstruation, or clothing that may come in contact with the lesions. Michael was fortunate that he could easily see the lesions at the tip of his penis. Often, however, the lesions could be located inside the penis or inside the vagina where direct visualization is not possible. Genital herpes is often accompanied by other systemic symptoms such as fatigue or a general sense of not feeling well, which can make arriving at an initial diagnosis difficult for health-care practitioners. Antiviral medication (e.g., valacyclovir) is typical first line drugs that are effective at controlling the severity of genital herpes symptoms and may shorten the duration of outbreaks. Michael's physician, however, was careful to emphasize that antiviral medication is not a cure for genital herpes; the sooner antiviral medications are begun, the more effective they can be at controlling the symptoms, and timing, of recurrent outbreaks. In contrast, suppression therapy is when antiviral medication is taken daily for several weeks or months as opposed to only when outbreaks are suspected or occur. Suppression therapy, then, is effective at controlling recurrent outbreaks when they become too frequent and minimizes the occurrence of genital herpes symptoms.

Genital herpes is contagious from an infected person to an uninfected sex partner, especially several days prior to the actual outbreak when viral shedding is at its highest. The proper and consistent use of condoms, especially when a person infected with genital herpes suspects an outbreak is imminent, will help minimize the transmission of the virus causing genital herpes. Sex partners of people diagnosed with genital herpes, then, should be alert for the development of similar symptoms within themselves and follow-up regularly with their health-care practitioner for screening tests and evaluation.

CASE 4: TINA

Tina is a 20-year-old college sophomore. She remained focused on her studies during her freshman year because it was her first time being away from home and she was determined to be successful in college. Additionally, Tina had broken up with her boyfriend prior to going away to college so she opted to dedicate her first year of school toward making new friends and getting good grades. Tina moved into a co-ed dorm where she quickly made new friends and became involved in numerous school activities. When Tina returned to school to begin her sophomore year she was introduced to a new male student who moved into her dorm. The two had many interests in common and eventually they began dating. As their relationship grew, Tina and her boyfriend became sexually active and occasionally had unprotected vaginal sex.

Tina was physically active and participated in various fitness activities like jogging and yoga. A few days following the end of her period, Tina was out for her usual jog when she noticed a burning, irritated sensation around her vagina. Suspecting her jog might be causing the irritation, Tina returned to her dorm. As she changed out of her work-out clothes, she noticed some musty smelling discharge on her underwear and thought the skin around her vagina looked reddened. Thinking she might have a yeast infection, Tina went to the local pharmacy and purchased a douche and over-the-counter fungal cream.

When Tina tried to use the douche, the burning and discomfort in her vagina increased. A long shower did little to decrease the irritation she felt or remove the musty odor. Applying the antifungal cream did little to calm the discomfort she felt. Following a restless night of sleep, Tina visited the student health service to have an evaluation by the nurse practitioner.

The nurse practitioner reviewed Tina's symptoms and took a thorough health history. She explained to Tina that she would need a physical examination with a pelvic exam so the nurse practitioner could better visualize the vagina and explore Tina's complaints. The nurse practitioner immediately noticed redness to the outside of Tina's vagina and the malodorous discharge. After inserting the speculum into Tina's vagina, the nurse practitioner saw copious amounts of white discharge inside and a reddened cervix. When the nurse practitioner took cultures from Tina's cervix, it began to bleed slightly. Based on Tina's symptoms and the physical findings the nurse practitioner discovered during the pelvic exam, the nurse practitioner made the presumptive diagnosis of trichomoniasis. Her diagnosis would be confirmed, then, if the cultures she took from Tina's cervix were analyzed in a lab and the microorganism, *T. vaginalis*, identified.

The nurse practitioner wanted to initiate antibiotic therapy quickly for Tina and not wait several days for the results of the cervical culture to arrive. The nurse practitioner prescribed a course of Flagyl, or metronidazole, a powerful antibiotic that successfully eliminates protozoans like *T. vaginalis*. The nurse practitioner carefully went over specific instructions for taking Flagyl with Tina, including the need to take the medication with food, finish the whole course of treatment even if she began to feel better, and to avoid alcohol use while taking the drug. The nurse practitioner encouraged Tina to speak to her boyfriend about coming to the student health service for an evaluation and possible treatment, and recommended HIV testing and screening for other STDs also. The nurse practitioner further advised Tina to use condoms with all episodes of sexual activity and to avoid sex until she completed the course of antibiotics and the symptoms disappeared. Lastly, the nurse practitioner confirmed a follow-up appointment at the student health service so she could reevaluate Tina, gauge the efficacy of the treatment plan, and discuss the results of the cervical cultures.

Analysis

Trichomoniasis is often a painful STD where the microorganism, *T. vaginalis* flourishes within the vagina. Tina experienced some of the most prominent initial symptoms of trichomoniasis: vaginal redness, vaginal discomfort or pain, and foul-smelling vaginal discharge. Because the symptoms arise suddenly and mimic other conditions initially such as a vaginal yeast infection, many women, like Tina, mistakenly try to treat the condition with over-the-counter preparations like douches or topical creams. Since the vagina is so irritated, over-the-counter treatments can cause increased discomfort and may promote additional growth of *T. vaginalis*.

The nurse practitioner was alert for the characteristic signs of trichomoniasis and knew that a pelvic exam was the only way to fully visualize the vaginal walls and the cervix. The reddened cervix that bled easily, then, is an additional hallmark of trichomoniasis when it involves inflammation of the cervix.

Trichomoniasis can lead to multiple complications for women, including the spread of the infection to involve the uterus or fallopian tubes, the formation of abscesses, or the development of pelvic inflammatory disease (PID). The nurse practitioner, then, opted to be proactive and quickly initiated antibiotic therapy that would be effective at eliminating *T. vaginalis*. Antibiotic therapy with Flagyl, however, can have multiple side effects and interactions so the nurse practitioner took additional time to educate Tina properly about the drug and its use. Since there was a strong presumption that Tina had trichomoniasis, there is also the potential she might have been exposed to other harmful, STD-causing microorganisms so additional STD and HIV screenings were indicated. Even if Tina completed the course of treatment and it was successful at eliminating the trichomoniasis, she could easily be reinfected by her boyfriend.

Screening, and possibly treating, sex partners of people diagnosed with trichomoniasis minimizes the opportunities for repeated reinfection. Sexual intercourse should be avoided until the treatment is completed and the symptoms disappear. The proper and consistent use of condoms when sexual activity resumes safeguards both partners from transmitting trichomoniasis or other STDs to each other.

CASE 5: KATIE

Katie is a 25-year-old woman who is a college graduate and works full time. She has been happily married to her husband for two years and they recently moved into their first home. Katie and her husband decided that the timing was ideal for them to begin starting a family. Realizing she had not had a physical or GYN exam in the past two years, Katie searched and found a midwife in her community and made an appointment to see her.

The midwife took time to carefully interview Katie about her medical, surgical, and sexual history. Katie admitted she had been sexually active with only three men in her life, including her husband. Kate reported that she and her husband have been mutually monogamous with each other for the duration of their relationship over the past five years, and that neither she nor her husband was ever diagnosed with an STD. The midwife noted, however, that Katie never received vaccines for human papillomavirus (HPV) during her teens or early twenties.

The midwife performed thorough physical and pelvic examinations on Katie. While Katie appeared healthy, the midwife took a Pap smear and other cultures from Katie's cervix to screen her for STDs and HPV. Before the appointment was over, the midwife provided Katie with information about proper nutrition in preparation for a future pregnancy and scheduled a follow-up appointment for Katie to review the test results.

When Katie returned for her follow-up appointment, the midwife informed her that, while her Pap smear was normal and no STDs were present, her screening test returned positive for HPV strains #16 and #18, the two strains that contribute the most to the development of cervical cancer. Because early detection of HPV is critical, the midwife recommended that Katie undergo a colposcopy that would allow magnified visualization of the cervix to determine if cervical damage, or disease, was present. Katie became concerned, then, about her ability to get pregnant in the future or the impact HPV could have on a baby. The midwife reassured Katie that while HPV is not curable there were measures that could be taken to minimize the effects of HPV. The midwife discussed the additional testing Katie would need and the follow-up testing that would be done at future visits. Last, the midwife reassured Katie that pregnancy would still be possible in the future and that, when it occurred, she would be followed closely by the midwife along with an obstetrician to keep her and her baby safe.

Analysis

Over 100 types of HPV, to date, have been identified. Forty of those strains have been identified to infect the genital areas. While several strains of HPV pose minimal risk and typically do not contribute to the development of cervical or anogenital cancers (e.g., strains #6 and #11), other strains such as #16 and #18 have been directly implicated to contribute to, or promote, the growth of cancers, especially within and around the cervix or endocervical canal. Most women, like Katie, often have no signs or symptoms that they have an internal infection with HPV. Genital warts within the genital area, if present, however, may be the only sign to alert a man or woman that they have HPV.

While there is no standardized testing for men to determine the presence of HPV, screening for HPV in women begins typically with a Pap smear around age 21. Since Katie had not had a physical or pelvic examination in over two years, the midwife decided wisely to initiate screenings for STDs and HPV while obtaining Katie's Pap smear. For most women, Pap tests are recommended currently every three years until age 65 if no abnormal cells are detected.

Abnormal Pap results or, like Katie, when HPV is detected warrant more frequent screening. For Katie, a colposcopy was recommended which would allow a more thorough examination of her cervix to identify any cancerous or suspicious lesions. A repeat Pap smear, then, typically occurs within 12 months to rescreen women for the continued presence of abnormal cells. While there is no cure for HPV currently, there are other measures that can be employed to minimize the harmful impact of HPV.

During colposcopy, a health-care practitioner can directly visualize any suspicious lesions and take a biopsy of the lesion for more detailed microscopic analysis in a laboratory. Cryosurgery, where a directed blast of liquid nitrogen or other gas carefully burns any suspicious lesions and allows new, healthy cervical tissue to regrow in its place, is another option for managing HPV lesions. Additionally, a LEEP (loop electrosurgical excision procedure) could be used to shave off thin layers of the cervix containing HPV lesions to remove traces of the harmful virus. These measures, while useful, can pose risks for women like Katie who wish to become pregnant in the future. Specifically, any procedure performed on the cervix can affect a woman's production of cervical mucus that is necessary to help sperm swim up into the reproductive tract and allow fertilization to occur, or the cervix can become weak. Cervical insufficiency, then, can make it difficult for women to carry a pregnancy to full term. Katie's midwife recognized these unique risks and created a plan to closely monitor Katie during any future pregnancies with prenatal care in collaboration with specialists.

Glossary

Anilingus: Contact with, and stimulation of, the anus using the mouth, tongue, or lips.

Cervical Insufficiency: A condition in which a pregnant woman's cervix begins to widen and thin before her pregnancy has reached full term.

Cervix: The narrow, cylinder-shaped structure that connects the vagina to the uterus.

Colposcopy: A cervical examination that uses a microscope to visualize the surface of the cervix to identify abnormal tissues or lesions.

Cunnilingus: Contact with, and stimulation of, a woman's genitals using the mouth, tongue, or the lips.

Cryosurgery: The use of extreme cold produced by liquid nitrogen (or argon gas) through a targeted blast or spray to destroy abnormal tissue.

Endocervical Canal: The passage, or tunnel, through the cervix that runs the length of the cervix into the uterine cavity.

Fellatio: Contact with, and stimulation of, a man's penis using the mouth, tongue, or lips.

Genital Tract: A term used to encompass the external and internal sex organs in both men and women.

Health-Care Practitioner: A licensed medical provider who can evaluate, diagnose, and treat various conditions or illnesses. Examples include physicians, nurse practitioners, midwives, or physician's assistants.

LEEP: Loop Electrosurgical Excision Procedure, or a procedure used to remove abnormal tissue from the cervix. It is done using a fine wire loop that has low voltage electrical current, which produces heat to remove thin layers of the cervix, especially after a colposcopy or cervical biopsy have confirmed an abnormal Pap result.

Pap Smear: Short for "Papanicolaou Smear," a test performed on a sample of cells from the uterine cervix to identify abnormal cells that may be indicative of cervical cancer.

Pelvic Exam: A procedure where a health-care practitioner examines the external structures of the vagina and rectum, then uses a speculum gently inserted into the vagina to visualize and examine the walls of the vagina and cervix. Often the examination is accompanied by a bimanual examination where the health-care practitioner uses two hands, one inside the vagina and one on the woman's abdomen, to gently palpate the uterus, fallopian tubes, and ovaries.

Pre-ejaculate: A clear, odorless fluid released by the male Cowper's gland during sexual arousal to provide lubrication for sexual activity (also known as "pre-cum").

Seminal Fluid: The fluid component of semen. Seminal fluid is produced by the prostate gland and seminal vesicles that provides a medium for sperm cells to travel outside a man's body.

Speculum: An instrument a health-care practitioner gently inserts into the vagina to separate the vaginal walls and allow visualization of and access to the vagina and cervix.

STD Screening: Samples of cells that come from blood, mouth, throat, inside the vagina, tip of the penis, rectum, or urine to detect the presence of harmful microorganisms that cause STDs.

❖

Directory of Resources

BOOKS AND ARTICLES

Ambrose, M., & Deisler, V. (2010). *Investigating STDs (sexually transmitted diseases): Real facts for real lives*. New York: Enslow Publishers.

Davis, K. K. (2015). *Let's talk about sex and STDs: A guide to prepare parents for "the talk."* Houston: Opportune Publishing.

D'Souza, A. H. (2014). *STDs*. North Charleston: CreateSpace Independent Publishing Platform.

Goodnough, A. (2016, October 19). Reported cases of sexually transmitted diseases are on the rise. *The New York Times*, p. A14.

ORGANIZATIONS

American Sexual Health Association (ASHA)

http://www.ashasexualhealth.org

The ASHA promotes the sexual health of individuals, families, and communities. ASHA specializes in communications outreach to the public, patients, press, providers, and policy makers by developing and delivering sensitive health information through many vehicles such as its website or publications. Above all, ASHA provides facts, support, and resources to answer questions, find referrals, join support groups, or get access to in-depth information about sexually transmitted infections and sexual health.

Centers for Disease Control and Prevention (CDC)

http://cdc.gov/std

The CDC provides a vast array of information on STDs. There are sections that report current STD statistics nationwide. The data contained within the CDC's website is updated regularly and is typically based on the latest scientific evidence. There are multiple links within the site to age-specific or disease-specific information in an easy-to-read and easy-to-navigate format.

Planned Parenthood

https://www.plannedparenthood.org/learn/stds-hiv-safer-sex

Planned Parenthood is a nonprofit organization that advocates for health care, health-care access, and reproductive care or choices for both men and women across the life span. Their website provides information on STD screening, access to care, and evidence-based education.

World Health Organization (WHO)

http://www.who.int

The WHO provides data and resources about STDs from an international perspective. The data contained within the WHO website is updated regularly and is based on the latest scientific data.

WEBSITES

AIDS.gov. https://www.aids.gov/hiv-aids-basics/

AIDSInfo. https://aidsinfo.nih.gov/

American Cancer Society, HPV and Cancer. https://www.fda.gov/forconsumers/byaudience/forwomen/ucm118530.htm

American College of Nurse Midwives. www.midwife.org

Gay Men's Health Crisis (GMHC). http://www.gmhc.org

Herpes. http://www.herpes.com/

I Wanna Know. http://www.iwannaknow.org/

Kids Health. http://kidshealth.org/en/parents/talk-child-stds.html

Medline Plus, The U.S. National Library of Medicine. https://medlineplus.gov/sexuallytransmitteddiseases.html

National Institutes of Health, National Institute of Allergy and Infectious Disease. https://www.niaid.nih.gov/diseases-conditions/std-research

STD GOV. https://www.std-gov.org/

U.S. Department on Health and Human Services, Office of Disease Prevention and Health Promotion. https://healthfinder.gov

U.S. Food and Drug Administration. https://www.fda.gov/forconsumers/ byaudience/forwomen/ucm118530.htm

WebMD. www.webmd.com

Your STD Help. http://www.yourstdhelp.com/std.faq.html

Youth Centered Health Design. http://yth.org/resources/youth-std-prevention/

Index

Anal sex, 12–13; and HIV, 61; and
STD risk, 12–13

Bacterial vaginosis, 19, 71–75; clue
cells, 73; definition, 71; diagnosis,
73; and pregnancy, 19; prevention,
74–75; signs and symptoms, 72;
transmission, 72; treatment, 74.
See also Pregnancy

Chancroid, 78–82; additional
considerations, 81; definition,
78–79; diagnosis, 80; and HIV,
80; prevention, 81–82; signs and
symptoms, 79–80; treatment, 81
Chlamydia, 19, 25–29; additional
considerations, 28; definition, 25;
diagnosis, 27; laboratory tests, 23;
and pregnancy, 19; prevention,
28; signs and symptoms, 26;
transmission, 28; treatment, 27.
See also Pregnancy
Circumcision, 129
Condoms, 13, 15, 21–22, 32, 35,
40–41, 45, 52, 55, 58, 70, 74,
78, 81, 87, 90, 93, 112, 119–20,
127–28; female condoms, 15,
70–71, 120; male condoms, 15, 70,
119–20
Condyloma lata, 48
Crabs, 98–101; and the care of
clothing, 100; diagnosis, 99;
prevention, 100; and sexual
activity, 101; signs and symptoms,
99; transmission, 99; treatment,
99–100; types of lice, 98. *See also*
Pubic lice; Sexual activity

Diaphragms, 35; douching and STDs,
120–21

Epididymitis, 18

Genital herpes, 35–41; additional
considerations, 39; definition,
35; diagnosis, 38; HSV–1, 36;
HSV–2, 36; and pregnancy, 17, 20,
39–40; prevention, 40–41; signs
and symptoms, 37–38; suppressive
therapy, 39; transmission, 37;

treatment, 38–39. *See also*
Pregnancy
Genital warts, 41–45; cryotherapy,
44; electrocautery, 43; definition,
41; diagnosis, 42–43; and HPV,
41; laser treatment, 44; liquid
nitrogen, 44; prevention, 44–45;
signs and symptoms, 41–42;
surgical removal, 44; transmission,
41; treatment, 43–44; vaccination,
45. *See also* HPV
Gonorrhea, 19, 29–33; additional
considerations, 31–32;
definition, 29; diagnosis,
30–31; laboratory tests, 23;
and pregnancy, 19; prevention,
32–33; signs and symptoms,
29–30; transmission, 29;
treatment, 31. *See also* Pelvic
inflammatory disease; Pregnancy

Hepatitis B, 19, 52–55; chronic,
54; definition, 52; diagnosis,
53–54; interferons, 54; laboratory
tests, 24; and the liver, 52, 55;
and pregnancy, 19; prevention,
54–55; signs and symptoms, 53;
transmission, 52–53; treatment, 54;
vaccine, 54–55
Hepatitis C, 20, 55–59; chronic, 58;
definition, 55; diagnosis, 57; and
the liver, 58–59; and pregnancy,
20; prevention, 58–59; signs and
symptoms, 56–57; transmission, 56;
treatment, 57–58
HIV (human immunodeficiency
virus), 59–71; AIDS, 65; ART
(antiretroviral therapy), 68–69;
CD-4 cells, 59–60; condoms and,
70–71; definition, 59; diagnosis,
65; disclosing test results, 67–68;
early stage, 64; frequency of
testing, 66–67; home tests, 66;
laboratory tests, 24; latent stage,

64–65; and pregnancy, 20, 61–62,
67; PrEP, 71; prevention, 69;
risk factors, 62–64; signs and
symptoms, 64–65; T cells, 59–60;
transmission, 60; treatment,
68–69
Homosexual sex, 14–15; men and,
14; preventive measures with, 15;
risks of, 14; women and, 14–15.
See also Condoms
HPV (human papillomavirus),
20, 82–85; abnormal cervical
cells, 84; and cervical cancer,
84; definition, 82; diagnosis,
83; genital warts, 84; laboratory
tests, 24; Pap test, 83–84; and
pregnancy, 20; prevention, 85;
signs and symptoms, 83; strains
of HPV, 82–83; transmission,
82; treatment, 84; vaccinations,
45, 85. *See also* Genital warts;
Pap test

Lice, 98–99; types of, 98–99. *See also*
Crabs, Pubic lice, Scabies
Lubricants, 13, 82, 121–22; and
prevention, 121–22. *See also*
Spermicides
Lymphogranuloma venereum
(LGV), 90–93; additional
considerations, 93; buboes,
92; definition, 90; diagnosis,
92; prevention, 93; signs and
symptoms, 90–92; stages, 91;
transmission, 90; treatment,
92–93

Molluscum contagiosum, 75
Mucopurulent cervicitis, 88–90;
additional considerations, 89;
definition, 88; diagnosis, 88–89;
and PID, 88; prevention, 90; signs
and symptoms, 88; treatment, 89.
See also Water warts

Oral sex: and STDs, 124–26; and chlamydia, 26; and syphilis, 47
Orgasm, 21–22; and STDs, 21–22

Pap test, 18, 23, 83–84; and HPV, 83–84
PID (pelvic inflammatory disease), 85–88; additional considerations, 87; definition, 85; diagnosis, 86; disease progression, 85–86; prevention, 87–88; signs and symptoms, 86; transmission, 85–86; treatment, 87
Pregnancy, 16–20, 39, 50, 61–62; and bacterial vaginosis, 19; and chlamydia, 17–18, 19; complications from STDs, 18; and gonorrhea, 18, 19; and hepatitis B, 19; and hepatitis C, 20; and herpes, 17, 20, 39; and HIV, 20, 61–62, 67; preconception screening, 18; and STDs, 16; and syphilis, 20, 50; and trichomoniasis, 18. *See also* Genital herpes; HIV
Pubic lice, 98–101

Scabies, 101–4; additional considerations, 103–4; definition, 101; diagnosis, 102; difference from crabs, 101; life span, 101; prevention, 104; signs and symptoms, 102; treatment, 102–3. *See also* Crabs
Sexual activity: and bacterial vaginosis, 72; and crabs, 101; and older people, 12; and young people, 11
Spermicides, 121–22; and STD prevention, 121–22. *See also* Lubricants
STDs (sexually transmitted diseases); bacterial, 9; and condom use, 112; definition, 3; diagnosis, 113–14; EPT (expedited partner testing),

115; fungal, 10; herbal or natural compounds, 118*t*; incidence, 4, 6–7, 11–12; laboratory tests, 22–23, 107–8, 110–11; in men and women, 10–11, 106–7; most common, 7; over-the-counter medications for, 117–19; parasitic, 9–10; partner treatment, 115–16; prevalence, 7; prevention, 119, 122–24; signs and symptoms, 105–7, 111–12; transmission during pregnancy, 18–21; types of, 8–10; and uncircumcised men, 128–29; untreated, 114–15; viral, 8; vs. STI, 4–6; when to be tested, 108–10; young people, 11. *See also* Condoms
Syphilis, 20, 45–52; additional considerations, 50; chancre, 46; definition, 45–6; diagnosis, 49–50; and HIV, 51; incidence, 47; laboratory tests, 23; latent or late, 48–49; and pregnancy, 20, 50; prevention, 51–52; primary, 47–48; stages, 47–49; transmission, 46–47; treatment, 50; treponemal test, 49–50; VDRL, 49. *See also* HIV

Transgender, 15–16; and STD risk, 15–16
Trichomoniasis, 21, 33–35; additional considerations, 35; definition, 33; diagnosis, 34; and pregnancy, 21; prevention, 35; signs and symptoms, 33–34; transmission, 33; treatment, 34–35

Water warts, 75–78; additional considerations, 77–78; definition, 75; diagnosis, 76; MCV–1, 75; MCV–2, 75; prevention, 78; signs and symptoms, 76; transmission, 76; treatment, 76–77. *See also* Molluscum contagiosum

Yeast infection, 93–98; balanitis, 96; *Candida albicans*, 94; diagnosis, 94–95; and douching, 95; and lactobacillus acidophilus, 96; and men, 96–98; prevention, 95; signs and symptoms, 94; and STDs, 93–94; treatment, 95. *See also* Yeast infection in men

Yeast infection in men, 96–98; diagnosis, 97; prevention, 97–98; symptoms of, 97; treatment, 97

About the Author

Paul Quinn, PhD, is a certified nurse midwife and women's health nurse practitioner with over two decades of acute-care experience in both nursing and midwifery practice within hospitals, clinics, and the private sector. An educator and women's health expert, he received his nursing diploma from Saint Vincent's Hospital School of Nursing, New York City, a Bachelor of Science in nursing from Pace University, New York City, and a Master of Science in nursing from the College of Mount St. Vincent, Bronx, New York. Later, he received an Advanced Certificate in Midwifery from the State University of New York-Downstate, Brooklyn, New York, and a Doctor of Philosophy from the City University of New York. His research track involves women's health issues, prenatal health and nutrition, and nursing workforce issues.